Connecting the dots....
between
development
and
behavior
in the learning environment,
home and community

Karen Hyche and Vickie Maertz

Connecting the dots..
First Edition 2024

ABOUT THE AUTHORS

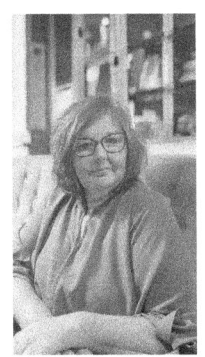

Karen Hyche, OTD, OTR, has dedicated over 25 years to specializing in pediatrics. She earned her Associate of Science Degree and completed the occupational therapy assistant program at the University of Alabama at Birmingham. Following this, she obtained her bachelor's degree in health care management from Birmingham Southern College and later pursued a master's in occupational therapy at Belmont University. In 2003, she completed her Doctorate in Occupational Therapy from Belmont University. Her clinic background includes public school system, early intervention as well as inpatient and outpatient psychiatric care. Karen opened The Hyche Center for Sensory & Motor Learning, a comprehensive pediatric clinic in Jasper, Alabama in 2015 where she continues to practice.

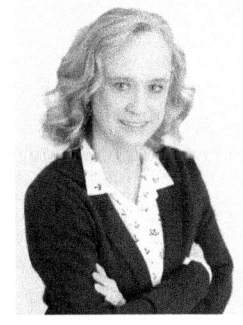

Vickie Maertz, OTD, OTR, has focused on pediatrics for over 25 years. She graduated from Belmont University in 2003, earning both a masters and a doctorate in occupational therapy. Before becoming an occupational therapist, she earn her associate degree as an occupational therapy assistant (COTA) from Houston Community College. Her clinical background includes early intervention, pediatric outpatient services, pediatric home health, and work within public and private school systems.

Vickie currently conducts professional-level lectures in the childcare industry, focusing on continuing education training regarding children with special needs. She lives in rural Texas with her husband, Travis, along with their grown children and grandchildren.

CONTENTS

Chapter 1   03
Connecting the dots

Chapter 2   07
Sensory System

Chapter 3   10
Sensory Processing Challenges

Chapter 4   27
Social Emotional

Chapter 5   34
Self Regulation & Co-regulation

Chapter 6   39
Attention Deficit Hyperactivity Disorder

Chapter 7   44
Autism

Chapter 8   52
Adverse Childhood Experiences

Chapter 9   55
Childhood Depression, Anxiety and Behavior

Chapter 10   64
Sleep Disorders and Nutrition

Chapter 11   72
Physical Activities and Play

Chapter 12   80
Treatment, Strategies and Activities

Resources, References   125

Chapter 1
Why Connecting the dots....

The goal of this book is to **enlighten caregivers, parents, teachers, and families** about not only sensory processing disorder and its impact on a child's behavior but also how so much more impacts a child's development in many different settings.

So together let's **connect the dots** on how sensory processing disorder (SPD) and other early childhood diagnoses can impact a child's behavior and development.

This comprehensive resource offers **practical strategies** to help caregivers, teachers, and families understand and support children with sensory differences.

Learn about the signs and symptoms of SPD, effective coping mechanisms, and how to create inclusive environments that foster growth and well-being in all children.

Visit us @

for more information on each chapter

CONNECTING THE DOTS

As parents and teachers your goal is to help children learn and develop skills to become independent adults. When children have difficulty learning, difficulty attending or just have many bad days, life becomes a struggle. Attempting to dissect the underlying issues can be complex. It is important to start at the beginning.

Foundational skills are the essential skills children need to build upon. The Pyramid of Learning was developed by occupational therapist Kathleen Taylor and special educator Maryann Trott. They utilized the Sensory Integration theorist, Jean Ayres', concepts to display the foundational skills that support academic learning.

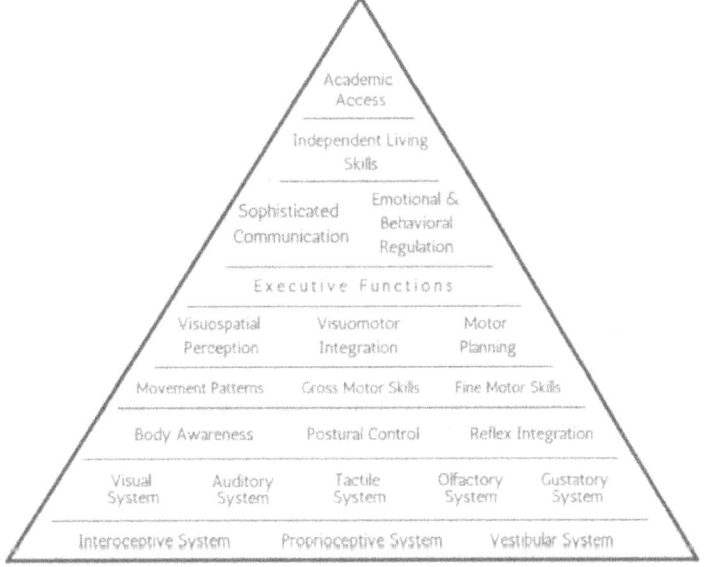

*Adapted from Taylor & Trott 1991; *The Alert Program*

What is that in more simplistic words....

At the very bottom are all the ways we sense the world around us: seeing, hearing, touching, smelling, tasting, moving, and knowing where our body is in space. These are our super cool senses!

The stronger these senses are, the sturdier the base of the pyramid. And guess what? A strong base helps the pyramid stand tall! That tall part is all about learning, like focusing in school, behaving well, and remembering things.

So, the more kids use their senses in a healthy way, the better they can learn and grow!

The Pyramid of Learning (Taylor and Trott)

The Pyramid of Learning, developed by occupational therapist Kathleen Taylor and special educator Maryann Trott, is a visual representation of the foundational skills necessary for optimal child development. It illustrates how sensory integration supports various developmental stages, from sensory systems to daily living activities.

Here's a breakdown of the Pyramid of Learning:

Foundation (Sensory Systems):
- **Tactile:** Touch
- **Vestibular:** Movement and balance
- **Proprioceptive:** Body position and awareness
- **Visual:** Sight
- **Auditory:** Hearing
- **Olfactory:** Smell
- **Gustatory:** Taste

Sensory Integration:
- **Registration:** The ability to receive and detect sensory information.
- **Organization:** The ability to process and interpret sensory information.
- **Modulation**: The ability to regulate sensory input and respond appropriately.

Sensory Motor Skills:
- **Fine motor skills:** Small muscle movements (e.g., writing, buttoning)
- **Gross motor skills:** Large muscle movements (e.g., walking, running, jumping)

Executive Functions:
- **Planning:** Organizing thoughts and actions.
- **Problem-solving: Finding solutions to challenges.**
- **Working memory:** Holding and manipulating information.
- **Attention:** Focusing and staying on task.

Daily Living Activities:
- **Self-care:** Dressing, eating, hygiene
- **Play and leisure:** Engaging in recreational activities
- **Social skills:** Interacting with others

Behavior and Academic Learning:
- **Behavior:** Managing emotions, following rules, and cooperating.
- **Academic learning:** Reading, writing, math, and other academic skills

The Pyramid of Learning emphasizes the importance of a strong foundation in sensory systems for supporting higher-level skills. By addressing sensory needs and building foundational skills, children can more effectively develop their executive functions, daily living skills, and academic abilities.

Relationship to Child Development:

Sequential Progression: The Pyramid of Learning emphasizes the sequential nature of child development. Children must master the foundational skills at the base of the pyramid before they can effectively develop the more complex skills at the top.

Interconnectedness: The levels of the pyramid are interconnected. For example, strong sensory integration skills are necessary for developing motor skills, which in turn impact cognitive development.

Holistic Approach: The Pyramid of Learning promotes a holistic approach to child development, recognizing the importance of addressing all aspects of a child's development, from sensory integration to social-emotional skills.

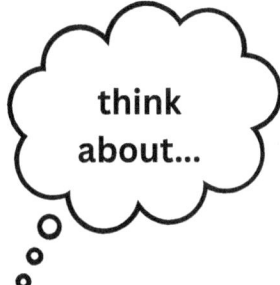

- Children should master foundational skills to reach their highest level of function.

- Without a strong foundation, learning can be difficult!

- There's more to sensory challenges than just being bothered by noise. Understanding the different senses and how they can impact the child is key.

- If children lack core strength, they tire easily and struggle to pay attention while sitting up straight.

Strategies can be found starting on page 80

Chapter 2
SENSORY SYSTEM

Scan QR code for more information on this chapter

Our sensory system, which is a component of the nervous system, comprises sensory receptors that detect stimuli from both the internal and external environment. This information is then processed to generate a response based on the sensory input. An example of this would be rain drops begin to fall as you are walking through the park. Your skin feels water, your eyes see water. That message is sent to your brain where your brain processes this information and then sends information for a physical response. An "acceptable" response would be to look in your bag for an umbrella or look for shelter. However, if the sensory information is identified as a threat or harmful, you may start screaming and asking for help.

Each sensory system has receptors that take the information to the brain to process.

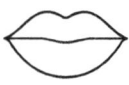 **Gustatory/Taste-** sense of taste. Taste buds allow the perception of taste, including sweet, salty, sour, bitter and umami. Buds are located on the back and front of the tongue and on the roof, sides and back of the mouth, and in the throat.

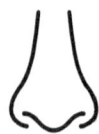 **Olfactory/Smell-** sense of smell. Smell information is sent directly to key brain regions involved in learning and memory. Our sense of smell is also directly linked to our sense of taste.

 **Auditory/Hearing-** sense of sound. The auditory system comprises outer structures, inner structures, and brain regions that process sounds to facilitate comprehension. These systems also assist in identifying the location and frequency of the sound.

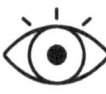 **Vision/Sight-** sense of sight. Our visual system detects shape, color, motion and depth. Six eye muscles around each eye allow visual focus, visual tracking and scanning.

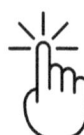 **Tactile/Touch-** sense of touch. The tactile system has two components; light touch and deep touch.
- The light touch pathway responds immediately and may set off a protective response.
- Deep touch pathways tells you where the person is touching you and how much pressure is being applied.

Touch is deeply connected to a sense of safety and security.

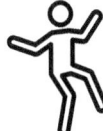 **Vestibular-** How we sense where are bodies are in space. The vestibular system provides the sense of balance and information about body position. Receptors for the vestibular system are located in the ear. Maintaining balance provides smooth movements and a sense of safety.

 **Proprioception-** sense of the way our body moves in space. Receptors are located in the muscles and joints. Input from this system allows movement and manipulation of objects without having to look at each body part. This system also provides information about force and heaviness.

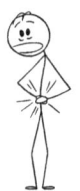 **Interoception-** sense of our internal regulation such as respiration, hunger heart rate and the need for digestion elimination. Interoceptive sensory processing plays a crucial role in higher-level cognitive functions, attention, memory, and the experience of self and time. Interoception is foundational to the experience and awareness of self and supports one's ability to trust that their body is relaying and regulating interoceptive sensation in a reliable way ([Oldroyd et al., 2019](#); [Chen et al., 2021](#)).

Many of the sensory systems work together. Here are some:

The Gustatory and Olfactory Senses:

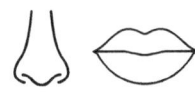 Gustatory and olfactory are distinct senses that collectively shape the sensation of flavor. Flavor, often referred to as the "taste" of food, encompasses smell, taste, spiciness, temperature, and texture. The majority of a food's flavor is derived from its smell; thus, losing the sense of smell significantly impacts flavor perception.

The Visual and Vestibular System:

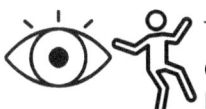 The visual and vestibular systems are interconnected through the vestibulo-ocular reflex (VOR). The VOR plays a crucial role in stabilizing the eyes during head movements, enabling visual focus during motion.

Interoception and Sensory Perception:

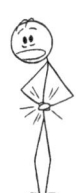 Interoceptive stimulation is detected by nerve endings in the respiratory and digestive mucous membranes. Interoception integrates vestibular and proprioceptive senses to regulate body perception. Well-regulated interoception helps individuals interpret proprioceptive and vestibular sensations effectively.

Sensory Milestones

Sensory Milestones in Children
Sensory processing is a child's ability to interpret and respond to sensory information from their environment.

Here are some key sensory milestones throughout childhood:
Infancy (0-12 months):
- **Visual:** Tracks objects with eyes, recognizes familiar faces, and develops depth perception.
- **Auditory:** Responds to sounds, turns towards noises, and recognizes familiar voices.
- **Touch:** Explores objects with their mouths and hands, shows sensitivity to textures.
- **Smell and taste:** Recognizes familiar smells and tastes, develops food preferences.

Toddlerhood (1-3 years):
- **Visual:** Recognizes colors, shapes, and patterns.
- **Auditory:** Follows simple instructions, understands basic concepts like "in" and "out."
- **Touch:** Shows increased sensitivity to textures, responds to touch cues.
- **Smell and taste:** Continues to develop food preferences, may become picky eater.

Preschool (3-5 years):
- **Visual:** Recognizes letters and numbers, can copy simple shapes.
- **Auditory:** Follows complex instructions, understands basic concepts like "before" and "after."
- **Touch:** Refines fine motor skills, can button and unbutton clothes.
- **Smell and taste:** Continues to develop taste preferences, may become more adventurous in food choices.

Elementary School (6-12 years):
- **Visual:** Reads and writes fluently, can identify details in pictures.
- **Auditory:** Can follow multi-step instructions, understands abstract concepts.
- **Touch:** Demonstrates refined motor skills, can write neatly and tie shoes.
- **Smell and taste:** Continues to develop sensory preferences, may become more sensitive to certain smells or tastes.

Remember, these are general milestones, and individual children may develop at different rates. If you have concerns about your child's sensory development, consult with a healthcare professional.

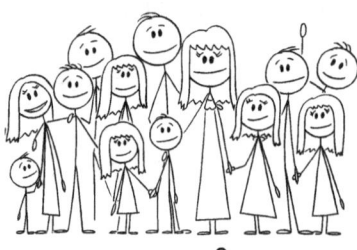

Chapter 3
SENSORY PROCESSING CHALLENGES

Scan QR code for more information on this chapter

We need to make sure that you understand that a majority of people/professionals call this Sensory Processing Disorder however.....

Sensory processing is not a disorder. The Diagnostic and Statistical Manual of Mental Disorders (DSM) is the handbook used by health care professionals in the United States and much of the world as the authoritative guide to the diagnosis of mental disorders. The DSM contains descriptions, symptoms and other criteria for diagnosing mental disorders.

There is mention of sensory deficits under diagnosis of ADHD, Autism and anxiety. However, there is not a specific diagnosis for sensory processing deficits. This is important for several reasons. Since it is not a diagnosis it is not a treatable diagnosis meaning insurance does not cover treatment of a disorder that does not exist. Insurance may provide payment for therapy for developmental delays, Autism, ADHD or other diagnosis. Therapy can then address the sensory issues that impact daily function.

Children ages birth up to a child's third birthday may benefit from early childhood intervention. Once a child reaches their third birthday they may qualify to receive services from their school district.

Research in this area has made significant gains. In 2013, UC San Francisco, researchers have found that children affected with SPD have quantifiable differences in brain structure, showing a biological basis for the disease that sets it apart from other neurodevelopmental disorders. The imaging detected abnormal white matter tracts in the SPD subjects, primarily involving areas in the back of the brain, that serve as connections for the auditory, visual and somatosensory (tactile) systems involved in sensory.

Sensory based challenges are real. These challenges have been divided into three distinct groups: **Sensory Modulation, Sensory-Based Motor and Sensory Discrimination**.

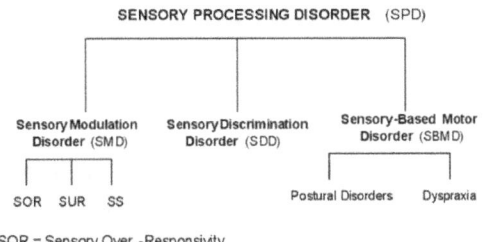

Graphic from Lucy J. Miller

Sensory Modulation is further divided in three categories;

- **Sensory Over Responsiveness-** Some kids feel things more intensely than others, like loud noises or itchy clothes. This can be frustrating and make them cry, have meltdowns, or get upset easily.

- **Sensory Under Responsiveness-** Children displaying under responsivity traits may appear reserved and introverted. While this behavior might not be obvious during infancy, it becomes more apparent as toddlers and older children are expected to engage in play with others.

- **Sensory Craving** -Children who have Sensory Craving exhibit a constant need for sensory stimulation and actively seek out sensory experiences, sometimes in ways that may not be socially acceptable. Behavior that may seem negative is often linked to sensory needs.

Each sensory system may be affected differently, for example a child may be craving tactile input but may be over responsive to auditory input.

Sensory Based Motor deficits are further categorized as:

- **Dyspraxia-** Individuals with Dyspraxia struggle with processing sensory information, leading to difficulties in planning and executing new motor actions. They may exhibit **clumsiness, awkwardness, and a tendency to break things**. Fine and gross motor skill challenges, **preference for sedentary activities**, and compensatory behaviors like verbalization or fantasy play are common.

- **Postural Disorder-** Individuals with Postural Disorders **struggle to stabilize** their body during movement or rest, affecting their ability to meet environmental demands or perform motor tasks. Good postural control enables reaching and resistance against force, while poor control leads to difficulty maintaining standing or sitting positions.

It is important to note that dyspraxia or developmental coordination disorder is a well established medical diagnosis.

Sensory Discrimination may also effect each sensory system differently.

Discrimination is the ability to interpret information. It allows you to compare various details, disregarding irrelevant information. Having a disorder of discrimination means struggling to interpret information or differentiate stimuli in affected sensory systems.

SENSORY MODULATION

Sensory modulation is our brain's ability to regulate its own activity. Our bodies and brains need to be able to filter out important sensory information and ignore irrelevant sensory information in order to formulate an adaptive response. This includes information from the five senses: sight, hearing, touch, taste, and smell. It also involves the vestibular sense (balance and movement) and the proprioceptive sense (body position and movement) along with interoception (ability to sense internal bodily states, such as hunger, thirst, pain, temperature, and emotions).

When sensory modulation is working well, the brain can effectively process and respond to sensory input, allowing for appropriate behaviors and reactions.
By interpreting sensory information properly, we are able to keep the body in a ready state. Our responses to stimuli are appropriate when we are regulated.

Individuals with modulation dysregulation do not interpert environmental information correctly and therefore their response is not "typical" or appropriate.

Individuals may have hypersensitivity or hyposensitivity to sensory inputs, impacting daily life and interactions. **Challenges** can affect social interactions, learning, and daily functioning.

Therapies like occupational therapy with sensory integration and creating supportive environments can help manage sensory modulation difficulties. Recognition and accommodation of sensory needs can improve well-being and promote inclusivity in society.

Here is a break down of Sensory Modulation

Over Responsive	Under Responsive	Craving/Seeking
Children who display **Over-Responsivity** often show a tendency to cry, have meltdowns, or react physically. They exhibit a greater sensitivity to sensory stimuli than the average population.	Children displaying **Under-Responsivity** traits tend to be reserved and introspective, especially evident as toddlers participate in social interactions and play.	Children with **Sensory Craving** have an increased longing for sensory stimulation, actively pursuing sensations, occasionally in ways that are socially inappropriate. What may appear as misbehavior is frequently linked to sensory requirements.

Over Responsive

> Children who exhibit **Over-Responsivity** are highly prone to crying, experiencing meltdowns, or reacting physically. They demonstrate a heightened sensitivity to sensory stimuli compared to the general population.

The following are examples for each system of what people who are over-responsive experience:

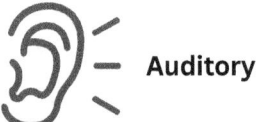

Auditory — Some people may find high-pitched sounds and frequencies irritating, voices might seem unusually loud, and sudden noises like slamming doors could startle them.

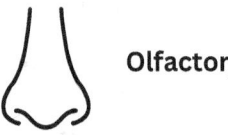

Olfactory — Some people experience a fight-or-flight response to sudden, strong smells, which might include gagging or vomiting. This can lead to them avoiding places with artificial scents like candles and air fresheners, and even disliking being around people who wear strong perfumes or colognes.

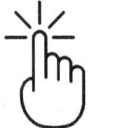

Tactile — Some children with sensory processing difficulties might experience clothing tags like needles piercing their skin, find gentle touches threatening, avoid baths due to water or washcloth discomfort, and participate less in messy art activities.

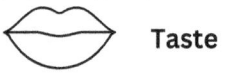

Taste — Picky eater with limited tolerance for taste, texture, or temperature variations; often prefers bland, room-temperature foods. Some children may crave extreme temperatures or strong flavors, enjoying heavily seasoned food with lots of condiments.

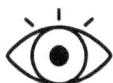 **Visual** — Some people experience distress from fluorescent lights, stress from flashing lights, and even sensitivity to colors.

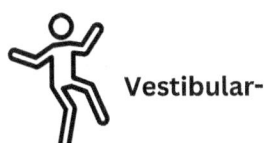 **Vestibular-** The child may have aversion to physical activity which makes exercise a challenge. Frequent bouts of carsickness limit their enjoyment of road trips.

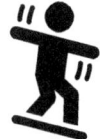 **Proprioception-** The child may find standing or walking uncomfortable and dislikes activities like jumping, hopping, or skipping.

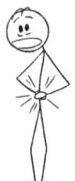 **Interoception-** Sensitive stomachs lead to frequent visits to the nurse's office, even for mild tummy aches.I

The child may

- refuse to participate in certain activities,
- become upset or sick when attempting to participate, or
- may push other children in response to stimuli.

The teacher and/or caregiver view behaviors as

- defiance,
- poor social skills, or
- the child being a bully.

This results in

- poor learning,
- poor self-esteem, or
- fewer friends.

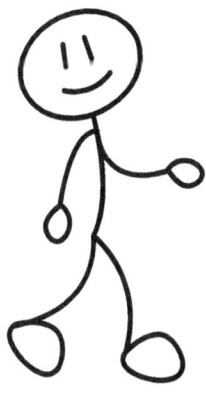

Under Responsive

> Children showing **Under-Responsivity** traits are reserved and introspective, more noticeable as toddlers engage in social interactions and play.

The following are specific examples for each system under-responsiveness may experience:

Auditory — Children with this combination might have difficulty processing sounds and speak loudly themselves.

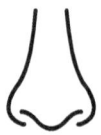
Olfactory — A student who might be seeking strong smells due to a lower sense of smell may sniff objects and people because they don't readily notice strong odors.

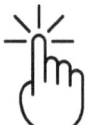
Tactile — Children may show a mix of reactions, including not noticing injuries (which can be dangerous), frequent touching of objects and people, and being oblivious to a messy face or wet clothes.

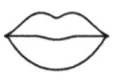
Taste — Children with reduced taste sensitivity might gravitate towards strong flavors to experience them more fully. Including a variety of flavors in their diet can help them explore different taste profiles.

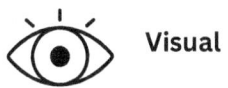 **Visual** Children may show a fascination with bright lights, lining up toys in specific ways, and spinning or visually stimulating objects. Also may also struggle with handwriting tasks like letter size, spacing, and pacing in an academic setting due to visual processing difficulties.

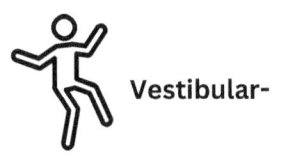 **Vestibular-** Children showing low movement awareness and high spinning tolerance may be unresponsive to vestibular stimulation. This can manifest as clumsiness, a fondness for spinning activities, difficulty coordinating movements using both sides of the body, and poor posture. In simpler terms, these children might seek out more movement to feel their bodies in motion and may be prone to falls due to a delayed awareness of their body's position.

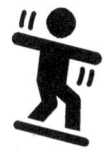 **Proprioception-** Despite enjoying running, they have a tendency to crash into objects. Their hand fatigues quickly while writing, causing them to press down hard on the pencil. Their enthusiasm can sometimes lead to pushing teammates a bit too hard, though it's always unintentional.

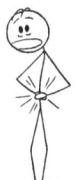 **Interoception-** May not often sense basic needs like breathing, hunger, or thirst, leading to challenges in performing daily tasks. This may result in slow potty training and development of enuresis. Additionally, individuals may not breathe or sweat properly due to a lack of awareness, potentially leading to interceptive discrimination dysfunction.

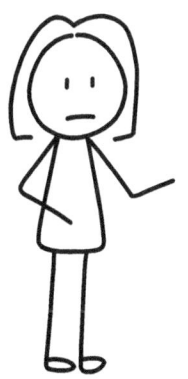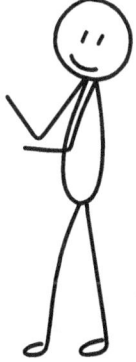

The child may
- not be responsive to injury,
- take longer to respond to commands, or
- lie around or prop up their head.

The teacher and/or caregiver may
- not recognize that the child is injured,
- view the child as being defiant, or
- view the child as lazy or uninterested.

This results in
- injuries,
- poor learning, or
- the child being left out

Craving/Seeking

> Children with **Sensory Craving** possess a increased desire for sensory stimulation, actively seeking out sensations, sometimes in socially inappropriate ways. What might be viewed as misbehavior is often connected to sensory needs.

The following are specific examples for each system who are sensory seeking may exhibit:

Auditory — Children with this combination might have difficulty processing sounds and speak loudly themselves.

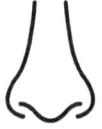

Olfactory — A student who might be seeking strong smells due to a lower sense of smell may sniff objects and people because they don't readily notice strong odors.

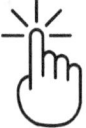

Tactile — Children may show a mix of reactions, including not noticing injuries (which can be dangerous), frequent touching of objects and people, and being oblivious to a messy face or wet clothes.

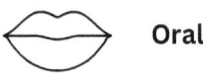

Oral — Children crave certain textures and flavors excessively. They frequently overstuff their mouth when eating, even to the point of gagging and will put anything in their mouth in search of oral input, such as chewing or crunchy sensations.

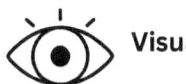 **Visual**
With a decreased sensitivity to visual stimuli, visual seekers crave intense visual input like lights, patterns, and moving objects. While they might appear to constantly seek stimulation, too much input can actually lead to overstimulation and a loss of focus.

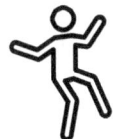 **Vestibular-**
Children often love to spin and rock and are often roller coaster enthusiasts. They appear to be in constant search for motion, which often leads to a diagnosis, be it accurate or of attention deficit hyperactivity disorder (ADHD)

 **Proprioception-**
They may seek out physical stimulation through bumping furniture, crashing onto cushions, roughhousing, or wrestling, and often prefer tight-fitting clothes.

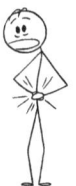 **Interoception-**
Children desire for intense sensory input may manifest as a constant need to move, rapid breathing, and seeking out feelings like a pounding heartbeat or a full bladder/bowel, even leading to a reluctance to eat or drink for fear of losing those sensations.

The child may
- not be able to sit still,
- hit or push others,
- chew on items or "fiddle" with items,
- turn the television or radio up or talk loudly, or
- run instead of walk

Teachers or caregivers may view the child as
- having attention deficit disorder (ADD), or
- being defiant

This results in
- poor learning experiences for the child.
- the child having difficulty maintaining, or
- the child disliking school.

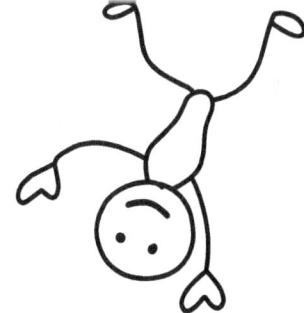

SENSORY DISCRIMINATION

Sensory discrimination disorder is defined by the Spiral Foundation as problems discerning an assigning meaning to qualities of specific sensory stimuli, poor recognition and interpretation of essential characteristics of sensory stimuli, and poor detection of differences or similarities in qualities of stimuli, for example, temporal/spatial qualities. Sensory discrimination may involve all senses but most commonly affects the tactile, vestibular, or proprioceptive senses and often co-occurs with dyspraxia and poor skill performance (Benson).

Sensory discrimination is all about your brain figuring out the details of what you experience through your senses. It's like having a built-in detective for your sight, touch, hearing, taste, and even balance!

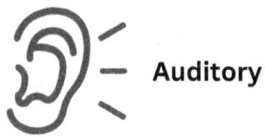
Auditory

Difficulty determining/interpreting characteristics of sensory stimuli that is heard. Ever struggle to tell the difference between words that sound similar, like "cat," "cap," and "pack"? This could be a sign of auditory discrimination disorder (ADD), which makes it difficult to distinguish the subtle details in sounds.

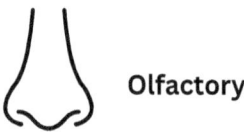
Olfactory

Think of it as your nose having trouble doing its detective work, making it hard to distinguish different smells. Does burnt toast ever smell like freshly baked cookies to you? This might be a sign of olfactory discrimination disorder!

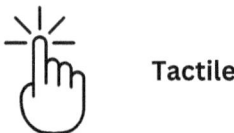
Tactile

Imagine closing your eyes and trying to identify a coin in your hand - is it a penny or a dime? Difficulty with this task could be a sign of tactile discrimination disorder. This means challenges in interpreting the details you feel through touch, including textures and shapes.

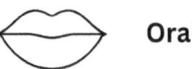
Oral

Imagine struggling to distinguish between sweet and sour, or bland and flavorful. This could be a sign of gustatory discrimination disorder, where your taste buds have difficulty recognizing different tastes. This can make enjoying food and distinguishing flavors a challenge.

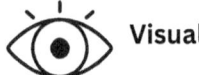
Visual

Imagine seeing a "P" but your brain might interpret it as a "Q." Or, a red apple appears green. This difficulty distinguishing visual details is called visual discrimination disorder (VDD).

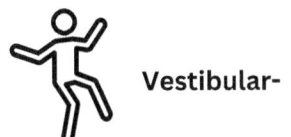 **Vestibular-** Challenges in interpreting sensory stimuli characteristics when the body moves through space or against gravity. Have you ever felt dizzy after spinning? Your vestibular system assists in perceiving your body's position and motion. Struggling to understand these signals is known as vestibular discrimination.

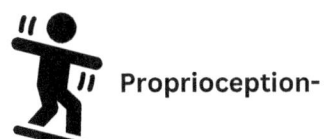 **Proprioception-** Struggling to interpret sensory stimuli related to muscle and joint usage. This sense acts as an internal body map, aiding in spatial awareness of body parts even without visual cues. For instance, proprioception enables tasks like touching your nose with your finger from behind your back! Challenges in comprehending these signals are known as proprioceptive discrimination difficulty.

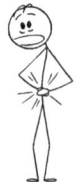 **Interoception-** Ever miss hunger cues or bathroom breaks? Our bodies constantly send messages about needs like thirst and fullness. Difficulty understanding these internal signals is called interoception discrimination difficulty. This can lead to confusion about bodily needs and even frequent stomachaches despite no physical problems.

Children with sensory discrimination deficits may drop items constantly. It may that they are doing this on purpose, but remember, they are not. Some children may difficulty putting steps of an activity together. You may have watched the student perfom activity the day before, but today they are unable to perform a similar activity. To a teacher is frustrating. It is to a child as well.

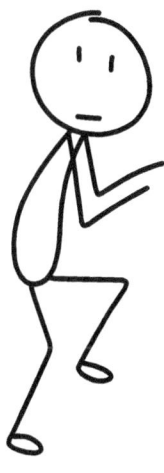

The child may
be clumsy, and
be rough or even break toys/pencils.

The teacher and/or caregiver may view the child as
being defiant,
being a bully, and
doing things intentionally to make him or her angry.

This results in
poor learning experiences for the child and
the child having few friends.

SENSORY BASED MOTOR

Sensory-Based Motor Disorders (SBMD):

Imagine struggling with balance, coordination, and activities like catching a ball or tying shoelaces. This could be a sign of SBMD. It happens when the brain has trouble processing information from the senses, making it difficult to plan and control movements. SBMD is different from conditions like Cerebral Palsy where there's a physical problem in the brain or nerves.

There are two types of sensory based-motor disorder:

Dyspraxia:

This is a specific type of SBMD that affects planning and carrying out new movements. It can make everyday activities like writing or getting dressed challenging. There are four steps involved in praxis. Here's how it works:

- **Ideation**: Difficulty thinking of the steps needed for a new task. For example, figuring out how to cut out a circle.
- **Planning:** the ability to plan how to complete task
- **Motor Planning:** Trouble organizing those steps in the brain.
- **Execution:** Difficulty actually carrying out the planned movements smoothly.

Postural Disorder:

People with postural disorder have trouble keeping their body steady, both when moving and staying still. This can make it hard to hold a good sitting or standing position, or to reach, push, and pull against objects.

Bilateral Integration and Sequencing
- One-sided weakness (not of neurological origin)
- Decreased arm swing when walking and/or running
- Possible head tilt
- Difficulty using both hands in the middle of the body
- Late emergence of a dominant hand
- Appearance of being lost or of being in a daze

Timing
- Human brain measures time continuously
- Requires a variety of human performance mechanisms (e.g., temporal processing; rhythm perception and production; synchronized motor behavior, etc.)
- Timing is essential to human behavior

Children with bilateral integration and sequencing difficulties have difficulty performing daily classroom tasks. They may not be able to hold their paper while writing or cutting.

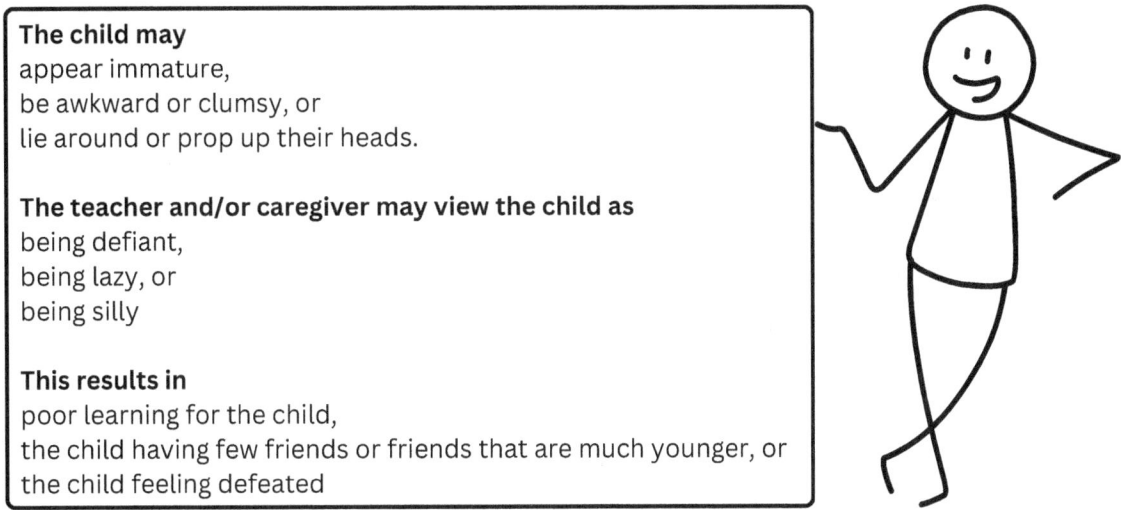

The child may
appear immature,
be awkward or clumsy, or
lie around or prop up their heads.

The teacher and/or caregiver may view the child as
being defiant,
being lazy, or
being silly

This results in
poor learning for the child,
the child having few friends or friends that are much younger, or
the child feeling defeated

You must keep in mind that a child may be sensory seeking in one area and sensory avoiding in another area. For example, a child may seeking in one area and typical in another area which can also change throughout the day.

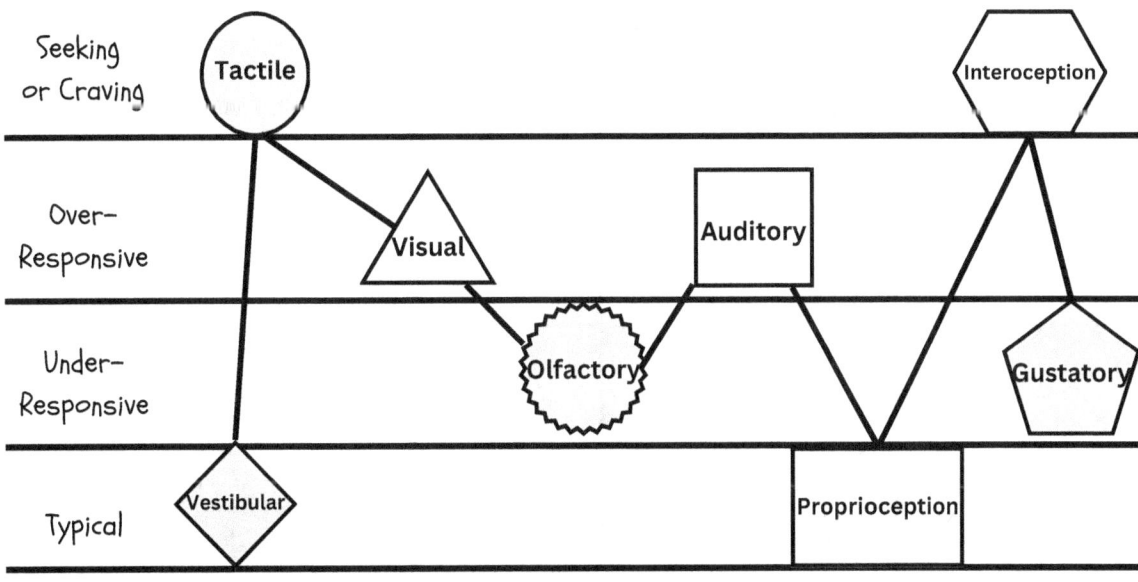

Summary of Sensory System

Sensory Modulation

Sense	Over Responsive	Under Responsive	Sensory Seeking
Auditory	• certain pitches in frequencies may be bothersome • voices may seem louder • easily startled	• does not respond to noises or name being called • may speak loudly	• difficulty coping with silence • makes noises • listens to loud music • prefers loud surroundings to quieter environments
Olfactory	• sudden odors can lead to fight or flight response • strong odors can lead to gagging or vomiting • Refuse to go to certain places or be around certain people due to odor	• May not respond to even very strong smells	• Chronically needs to smell things • prefers environments that are always filled with fragrances
Tactile	• Tags seem like needles piercing their skin • A simple touch can be perceived as a threat • Poor hygiene due to dislike to fill of water and washcloth • Poor participation in activities	• Fails to react to tactile experiences (decrease self protection) i.e. injuries • May constantly touch objects and people • Unaware of messy face, wet clothes, etcetera	• Likes playing with sand and muck • May run hands or fingers across walls, railings, and other objects in the environment • Constantly touch other people
Vision	• Fluorescent lights may be distressing • new line Flashing lights may be stressful • sensitivity to colors	• Stares into bright light • lining up toys/ uobjects • be overly drawn to spinning or stimulating objects	• May surround self with vivid, flashing, or blinking lights • stares at fast moving objects • May also stare directly at lights

Summary of Sensory System

Sensory Modulation

Sense	Over Responsive	Under Responsive	Sensory Seeking
Vestibular	• Sudden change in head position may cause distress • Avoid physical activities • Car sickness • Fear of heights	• Does not seem to notice when they are being moved. • Does not register movement effectively enough to decipher when dizzy. • May not notice when falling, which can result in decreased protective	• Often love to spin and rock, and often is a roller coaster enthusiast. • Constant search of motion often leads to a diagnosis, be it accurate or not, for attention deficit hyperactivity disorder.
Gustatory	• Picky eater; may only eat specific textures or temperatures of foods	• Does not have food preferences • Enjoys spicy or sour foods	• Constantly eating or drinking • Likes chewy and crunchy foods • Overstuffs mouth
Proprioceoption	• Avoids movement • Appears rigid or tense	• Poor body awareness • Poor posture • Low energy	• Crashes and into things • Loves contact sports or activities
Interception	• May use bathroom frequently • May over eat • Distressed when hot or hungry	• May not be aware of hunger or thirst • May not notice need to go to bathroom	• May over eat or avoid eating • May avoid going to bathroom

Sensory modulation is often dificult to understand because a child can present with different symptoms or even without symptoms depending on the day. Our sensory responses are based on our physical and emotional well-being. A child who may not feel well or who may not have slept well could have a more difficult day whereas the same child, having slept well, may exhibit no or minimal signs of SPD the next day. You must also keep in mind a child may be sensory seeking in one area and sensory avoiding in another area. For example a child may demonstrate the following symptoms.

Summary of Sensory System

Sensory Discrimination

Sensory System	Behavior
Prioprioception	- Has great difficulty grading movement - Rough with peers - Walks toe walks - Chews on shirtsleeve and/or grinds teeth - Frequently bumps into objects - May fall down more than peers of the same age
Tactile	- Very "touchy-feely," often inappropriately touching objects or people - Sloppy (clothes are twisted, does not notice food left on their face following a meal) - High pain tolerance - Difficulty locating or naming items with the eyes closed - Drops items frequently - Drools past expected age - Mouths objects past expected age - Poor fine motor skills - Poor speech articulation
Vestibular	- poor awareness of movement of body in space (gets disoriented easily) - knows he's falling, but can't tell which way and can't protect himself
Dyspraxia	- Difficulty cutting with scissors - Difficulty performing various fine motor activities, such as zipping and buttoning clothing without looking - Difficulty with dressing and handwriting - Have a hard time navigating through crowded hallways or noticing obstacles before collision - Unable to use what has been previously learned to help with new tasks - Experience anxiety around moving through space or moving up or down stairs - May often over or under extend muscles to perform a task, causing one to break things or drop them

Summary of Sensory System	
Sensory Based Motor	**Behavior**
Dyspraxia: Bilateral integration and sequencing	- One-sided weakness (not of neurological origin) - Decreased arm swing when walking/running - Possible head tilt - Difficulty working at the mid line of the body - Difficulty weight shifting - Late emergence of a dominant hand - May appear lost or in a daze
Postural Based	- Frequently drool and have difficulty keeping things in your mouth - Poor posture while sitting or standing - Sit in awkward positions, like over the edge of a seat - Often lean head forward onto hands, arms, or other objects when working at a desk or eating

CHAPTER 4
SOCIAL EMOTIONAL

Scan QR code for more information on this chapter

Parents and caregivers play the biggest role in social/emotional development because they offer the most consistent relationships for a child. Consistent experiences with family members, teachers and other adults help children learn about relationships and explore emotions in predictable interactions.

Social Emotional developmental domain encompasses five specific areas: **self awareness, self-management, social awareness, relationship skills** and **responsible decision making.**

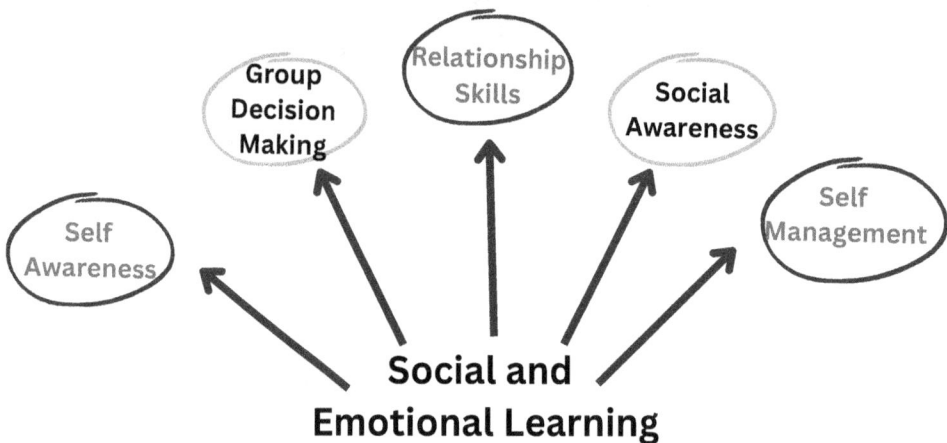

Social development is all about how children learn to interact with the world around them, both with other people and in understanding their place within that world. It's a gradual process that starts from birth and continues throughout childhood.

Self-awareness
A crucial skill is recognizing and understanding your emotions, thoughts, and values, and comprehending how they influence your actions. It involves evaluating your strengths and acknowledging that abilities and intelligence can be developed. Key skills include:

- identifying emotions
- self-perception
- recognizing strengths
- self-confidence
- self-efficacy

Self-management
This is the ability to manage and regulate your emotions and behavior, including managing stress, controlling impulses and keeping yourself motivated. The main skills include:

- impulse control
- stress management
- self-discipline
- self-motivation
- goal-setting
- organizational skills.

Social awareness
This is the ability to understand and empathizes with people from a range of diverse backgrounds, and to understand social and ethical norms of behavior. The main skills include:

- perspective-taking
- empathy
- appreciating diversity
- respect for others.

Relationship skills
These involve the ability to develop and maintain healthy and positive relationships with others. They include the ability to communicate clearly, listen, cooperate, resist peer pressure and negotiate conflict. The main skills include:

- communication
- social engagement
- relationship building
- teamwork.

Responsible decision-making
This is the ability to make informed and responsible decisions about personal behavior and social interactions with others, based on adherence to ethical standards, safety concerns and social norms. The main skills include:

- identifying problems
- analyzing situations
- solving problems
- self-evaluation
- self-reflection
- ethical responsibility.

Here is an overview of the **social-emotional milestones** that children usually achieve at various ages.

Newborn to 6 Months
- Develops basic trust and attachment with caregivers
- Begins to smile and coo in response to interaction
- Shows distress when separated from caregivers

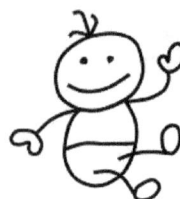

6 to 12 Months
- Shows separation anxiety when caregivers leave
- Expresses a wider range of emotions, such as happiness, sadness, and anger
- Begins to interact with others through gestures and sounds

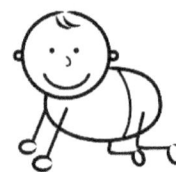

12 to 18 Months
- Shows more independence and exploration
- Plays simple games like peek-a-boo
- May experience stranger anxiety
- Begins to understand the concept of "no"

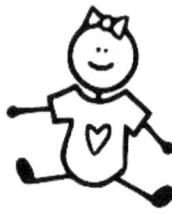

18 to 24 Months
- Shows more empathy and concern for others
- Engages in parallel play, playing alongside other children but not necessarily with them
- Begins to assert independence and may have frequent temper tantrums
- Uses simple words and phrases to express emotions

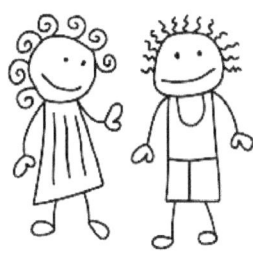

2 to 3 Years
- Engages in more pretend play
- Begins to cooperate with others in play
- Shows a wider range of emotions and is able to talk about them
- Starts to toilet train

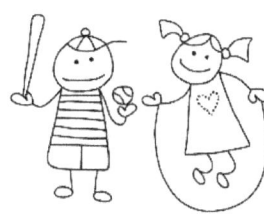

3 to 4 Years
- Shows more complex emotions, such as jealousy and pride
- Plays more cooperatively with others
- Can follow simple rules
- Starts to dress themselves

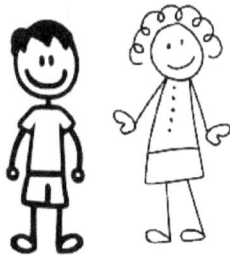

4 to 5 Years
- Shows increased self-awareness and self-esteem
- Understands the concept of sharing and taking turns
- Can express their feelings more clearly
- Begins to develop friendships

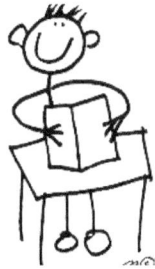

5 to 6 Years
- Shows more complex emotions, such as guilt and disappointment
- Can regulate their emotions more effectively
- Plays cooperatively in group games
- Can follow multiple rules

It's important to remember that every child develops at their own pace. If you have any concerns about your child's social-emotional development, talk to their doctor.

Numerous factors can influence the social-emotional development of young children, which can be categorized into three main groups:

Environmental Risk Factors:

- **Living in Unsafe Communities:** Exposure to violence, poverty, or instability can lead to chronic stress, impacting emotional regulation and social interactions.

- **Low-Quality Childcare:** Inadequate environments or insensitive caregivers in daycare settings can limit social learning and emotional expression.

- **Limited Resources:** Challenges in overall development may arise from insufficient access to healthcare, nutritious food, or educational opportunities.

Family Risk Factors:

- **Mental Health Issues in Parents:** Parental depression, anxiety, or substance abuse can create an unstable and stressful home environment. If a mom or dad is struggling with depression, anxiety, or drugs, it can make the home environment feel tense and unpredictable. This can make it hard for kids to feel secure and learn healthy emotional responses.

- **Attachment Problems:** Insecure attachment due to neglect or abuse can hinder the ability to form trusting relationships. Thus, if a child wasn't properly cared for as a baby, they might have trouble forming trusting bonds with others as they grow and mature. This can make them seem withdrawn or act out.

- **Family Violence:** Witnessing violence between family members at home can disrupt a child's sense of security, impacting good social skills and emotional regulation.

Within-Child Risk Factors:

- **Developmental Delays:** Challenges in communication, social interaction, or emotional understanding are common for children with that experience developmental delays.

- **Mental Health Conditions:** Social settings and emotional expression may be overwhelming or difficult to understand when paired with anxiety, ADHD, or autism spectrum disorder.

- **Serious Health Issues:** Social isolation and difficulty managing emotions can be experienced due to chronic health problems causing pain or discomfort. If a child is often sick or in pain, it can make them feel isolated and withdrawn. This can make it hard for them to learn social skills and manage their emotions.

It is essential to recognize that these factors often intersect. For example, poverty can heighten the risk of family violence, leading to attachment issues.

Early intervention is vital. If you observe any difficulties in your child's social-emotional development, consult their pediatrician or a child development specialist for support and resources to enhance your child's well-being.

Typical and Non-Typical Behaviors in Children

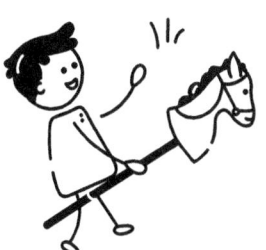

Typical behaviors are those that are considered normal and expected for a child's age and developmental stage. They align with general social, emotional, and cognitive milestones.

Non-typical behaviors are those that deviate from the expected norms, often indicating underlying concerns or developmental challenges.

Here's a general overview of typical and non-typical behaviors:

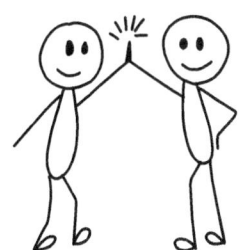

Typical Behaviors:
- **Social:** Plays with peers, shares toys, follows rules, shows empathy.
- **Emotional:** Expresses a range of emotions, manages feelings, understands social cues.
- **Cognitive:** Learns and develops new skills, follows instructions, solves problems.
- **Behavioral:** Engages in appropriate activities, avoids harmful behaviors.

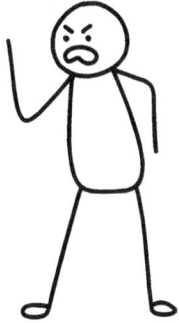

Non-Typical Behaviors:
- **Social:** Difficulty interacting with peers, isolation, aggression.
- **Emotional**: Excessive anxiety, depression, or mood swings.
- **Cognitive:** Delays in language, motor skills, or academic achievement.
- **Behavioral:** Challenging behaviors, such as tantrums, aggression, or self-harm.

It's important to note that this is a general overview, and individual children may exhibit variations. If you have concerns about your child's behavior, it's recommended to consult with a healthcare professional for further evaluation.

Expected Behaviors in Children

Expected behaviors in children can vary depending on age, cultural background, and individual personalities. However, there are some general guidelines that most societies and cultures agree upon.

General Behavior Expectations in Children:

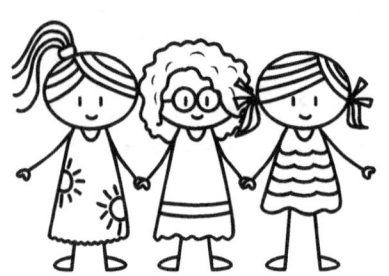

- **Respect:** Children should respect authority figures, peers, and property.
- **Cooperation**: They should be able to work well with others and share.
- **Responsibility**: Children should take responsibility for their actions and belongings.
- **Self-control:** They should be able to manage their emotions and impulses.
- **Honesty:** Children should be truthful and avoid lying.
- **Kindness:** They should treat others with kindness and compassion.

Age-Specific Expectations:

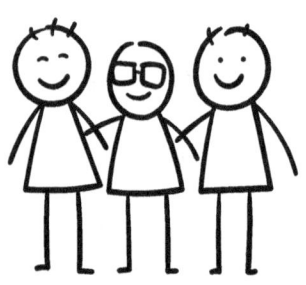

- **Toddlers (1-3 years):** May exhibit tantrums, but should generally be able to follow simple instructions.
- **Preschoolers (3-5 years):** Should be able to share toys, take turns, and follow rules.
- **Elementary school (6-12 years):** Should be able to complete tasks independently, follow complex instructions, and participate in group activities.

Remember, children are still learning and developing, so it's important to be patient and understanding. If you're concerned about your child's behavior, consider talking to a teacher, counselor, or pediatrician.

CHAPTER 5
SELF REGULATION & CO-REGULATION

Scan QR code for more information on this chapter

People tend to think of Self Regulation first however a child learns to Self Regulate after they experience Co-regulation.

Self-regulation is a person's ability to adjust and control their energy level, emotions, behaviors and attention. Appropriate self regulation is when a person is able to adjust and control themselves in ways that are socially acceptable.

Self-regulation isn't innate; it's a skill children develop through interactions with trusted adults. Co-regulation, a process that begins in infancy, involves warm, consistent, and responsive adult interactions that help shape a child's self-regulation abilities.

Developing self-regulation is a journey, not a destination. Celebrate the small victories along the way, and provide lots of love and support as the child hones these essential life skills. With time, patience, and practice, the child will learn to use their "toolbox" effectively, setting them up for a lifetime of success and well-being.

Self-regulation involves individuals managing their behavior independently. It offers various advantages for children, including learning to handle challenging emotions and navigate stressful circumstances effectively. Additionally, self-regulation empowers children to feel in control of their emotions, promoting a sense of calm and stability.

Self-regulation in young children involves learning to **manage their emotions and reactions** in a healthy manner. It marks the distinction between a toddler having a complete meltdown and a kindergartener being able to self-soothe to some extent.

Self-regulation is nurtured and developed through **co-regulation**, where adults and children collaborate towards a common goal, such as addressing stress-related upsets in various aspects and restoring balance. With time and consistent practice, co-regulation transitions into the child's self-regulation. During the early years, the brain's adaptability allows for changes in its architecture based on the quality and regularity of co-regulation experiences, thus enhancing the ability for self-regulation.

Self-regulation isn't just about following directions, like sitting still and being quiet. Imagine a child who's feeling jittery and really wants to wiggle or talk. That's different from a child who's calm and focused, with their feelings, thoughts, and actions all in check.

Just like adults, kids have good and bad days with self-regulation. It's not something they have all the time or not at all. But if a child seems to be struggling a lot more than usual, it might be a sign they're feeling very stressed or had something scary happen.

> **Here's a breakdown:**
>
> **What it is:** Self-regulation is a skill that helps young children understand their feelings, control their impulses, and behave appropriately.
>
> **Why it's important:** Strong self-regulation skills set children up for success in school, friendships, and overall well-being. It helps them focus, deal with frustration, and navigate social situations.

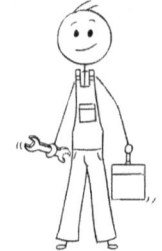

Imagine self-regulation as a toolbox for your child. This toolbox has many helpful things inside!

- **Impulse control:** This helps your child stop and think before they act. Like holding back from grabbing that last cookie!

- **Managing emotions:** This helps your child calm down when they're mad or sad, and cheer up when they're feeling low.

- **Self-guidance:** This helps your child figure out what to do next, like solving a problem or making a good choice.

These are just a few of the tools in the box. There are even tools for babies, like learning when they're hungry or tired. But the most important ones are the emotional and thinking tools. These help kids understand their feelings and thoughts, and then act in a positive way.

Self-regulation is super important because it helps kids with everything from making friends and learning in school to feeling happy and healthy. It's like a superpower that helps them navigate life!

And just like any superpower, self-regulation takes practice to master. Parents and caregivers can play a key role in helping children develop these skills by modeling good self-regulation themselves. When kids see adults managing their emotions, making thoughtful decisions, and handling stress calmly, they learn to do the same.

Here are some tips for nurturing self-regulation in your child:

- **Create a Routine:** Consistent schedules provide a sense of security and predictability, which can help kids manage their impulses and emotions better.

- **Teach Problem-Solving Skills:** Encourage the child to think through solutions when they encounter a problem. Ask open-ended questions like, "What do you think we should do?" or "How can we fix this?"

- **Encourage Expression:** Let the child know that it's okay to feel a range of emotions. Encourage them to talk about their feelings and validate their experiences.

- **Practice Mindfulness:** Simple mindfulness exercises, such as deep breathing or a few moments of quiet reflection, can help children learn to stay calm and focused.

- **Praise Effort, Not Just Success:** Recognize and celebrate the effort your child puts into managing their emotions and making good decisions, even if things don't always go perfectly.

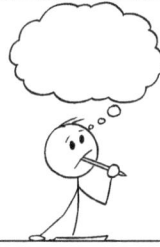

Think about:
Babies cry to tell us they need something. They might be hungry, tired, or uncomfortable. When a baby is really upset, it's hard for them to calm down on their own. This is where caregivers come in!

Here's how caregivers help:

Calming the baby: By talking softly, picking them up gently, and figuring out what's wrong, caregivers help babies feel safe and loved. This back-and-forth is called co-regulation. It's like a game of catching: the caregiver catches the baby's feelings and helps them calm down.

Building emotional skills: As babies experience co-regulation, they learn how to manage their own emotions. They start to understand that even when they're upset, things can get better. This is like building a special brain path for handling feelings.

Learning and emotions go hand-in-hand. For example, a baby might cry loudly at first when their caregiver leaves the room. But if the caregiver always comes back quickly, the baby learns to wait a bit. They know help is on the way, even if they can't see it yet. Over time, babies can even learn to soothe themselves, like sucking on a thumb or rocking back and forth.

Co-Regulation

Co-regulation supports children in acquiring positive self-regulation skills. By observing adults manage their emotions, children can learn to do the same, fostering a sense of safety. Feeling secure enables children to remain calm and composed.

Co-regulation is essentially how young children learn to regulate their emotions by **observing and engaging with the adults** in their environment. It's like a synchronized dance where your calmness helps your child calm down too.

Co-regulation involves connecting with a distressed child, assessing their needs, and helping them calm down. Before assisting a child, adults should be aware of their own emotional skills and limitations. Emotions are often contagious, whether positive or negative.

Co-regulation requires a warm, responsive relationship with children, along with clear structure and limits. Consistent, predictable routines with clear expectations and consequences benefit children.

When a child experiences strong emotions, a **co-regulation** response will vary based on the child and situation.

Building the Foundation: Co-Regulation and Emotional Regulation

Newborns lack the ability to manage their emotions independently. During the first three years, they rely on caregivers to soothe and calm them. This process, called coregulation, involves adults responding sensitively to babies' cries, facial expressions, and body language. Through touch, voice, and gaze, caregivers help the child cope with strong emotions.

Co-Regulation paves the way for self-regulation, the ability to manage emotions, thoughts, and behaviors independently. Consistent, responsive interactions with trusted adults are crucial for developing self-regulation. These adults, including family and caregivers, provide comfort and soothing, laying the foundation for emotional well-being.

Emotional regulation is a cornerstone of healthy development. Studies show that children with good self-regulation tend to experience better health, higher incomes, and greater life satisfaction later in life. The first three years are particularly critical for building this foundation as young children move from relying on coregulation to managing their own emotions increasingly.

Here's a breakdown of co-regulation in young children:

- **Foundation for Self-Regulation:** Co-regulation serves as the basis for self-regulation, enabling children to manage their emotions. Through co-regulation with a nurturing adult, kids develop healthy coping mechanisms for stress and intense emotions.

- **Emotional Support:** Co-regulation involves being present for your child during emotional moments, acknowledging their feelings, and assisting them in finding ways to relax.

- **Calming Techniques:** Through co-regulation, you can introduce coping mechanisms like deep breathing or taking breaks. As your child grows, they can start using these techniques independently.

Encouraging **self-awareness and emotional intelligence** is also crucial. Teach the child to recognize their feelings and understand what triggers their stress. You can use tools like emotion charts or journals to help them articulate their emotions.

Remember:
- **Consistency and Routine:** Establishing a predictable routine can provide a sense of security and stability. Regular schedules for meals, bedtime, and activities can help reduce anxiety and make transitions smoother.

- **Positive Reinforcement:** Celebrate small successes and efforts. Positive reinforcement can motivate your child to keep practicing self-regulation techniques. This could be in the form of verbal praise, stickers, or extra playtime.

- **Create a Calming Environment**: Designate a quiet space in your home where your child can retreat when they need to calm down. This area can include comforting items like soft pillows, blankets, or a favorite stuffed animal.

- **Physical Activity:** Encourage regular physical activity, which can help reduce stress and improve mood. Activities like yoga, dancing, or simply playing outside can be very beneficial.

Remember, every child is unique, and what works for one may not work for another. Patience and persistence are key. By consistently supporting and guiding your child in these practices, you will help them develop essential skills for managing their emotions and stress effectively.

Strategies can be found starting on page 80

CHAPTER 6
Attention Deficit Hyperactivity Disorder

Scan QR code for more information on this chapter

Attention Deficit Hyperactivity Disorder has had numerous different labels over the past century, including hyperactive child syndrome, hyperkinetic reaction of childhood, minimal brain dysfunction, and attention deficit disorder (with or without hyperactivity). In the DSM-5 Text Revision published in 2022 regarding the diagnostic entity of Attention Deficit/Hyperactivity Disorder (ADHD) there were some changes. It is stated in the DSM-5 TR that ADHD is a persistent pattern of inattention and/or hyperactivity-impulsivity that interferes with functioning or development.

Russell Barkley is a leading researcher and educator in the field and is internationally recognized authority on attention deficit hyperactivity disorder (ADHD/ADD) in children & adults. He defines attention-deficit hyperactivity disorder (ADHD) as the current term for a specific developmental disorder seen in both children and adults. It is comprised of deficits in behavioral inhibition, sustained attention and resistance to distraction, and the regulation of one's activity level to the demands of a situation (hyperactivity or restlessness).

Attention deficit hyperactivity disorder (ADHD) is a persistent condition that can affect both boys and girls, although boys are diagnosed more frequently. There's no single test for ADHD, but diagnosis relies on a careful evaluation.

While symptoms may appear in early childhood, the Diagnostic and Statistical Manual of Mental Disorders (DSM-5) acknowledges the difficulty of distinguishing them from typical behaviors in children under age 4.

According to the DSM-5 TR there are three presentations of ADHD:

- Combined type: Inattention and hyperactivity/impulsivity
- Predominately Inattentive without hyperactivity/impulsivity
- Predominately Hyperactivity/Impulsivity without inattention

The DSM-5 TR then goes into it a little deeper by defining if subtype is:

•**Mild:** Few, if any, symptoms in excess of those required to make the diagnosis are present, and symptoms result in no more than minor impairments in social or occupational functioning.

•**Moderate:** Symptoms or functional impairment between "mild" and "severe" are present.

•**Severe:** Many symptoms in excess of those required to make the diagnosis, or several symptoms that are particularly severe, are present, or the symptoms result in marked impairment in social or occupational functioning

Understanding and Defining the Components of ADHD:

The criteria of symptoms for a diagnosis of ADHD: In making the diagnosis, children still should have **six or more symptoms** of the disorder. In older teens and adults the DSM-5 states they should have at **least five symptoms.**

The DSM- 5TR requires an individual's symptoms to be present prior to age 12, compared to 7 as the age of onset in DSM-IV. Substantial research published since 1994 found no clinical differences between children with earlier versus later symptom onset in terms of their disorder course, severity, outcome, or treatment response. Other criteria for diagnosing children with ADHD remain unchanged.

Inattentive presentation:

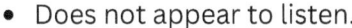

- Fails to give close attention to details or makes careless mistakes.
- Has difficulty sustaining attention.
- Does not appear to listen.
- Struggles to follow through on instructions.
- Has difficulty with organization.
- Avoids or dislikes tasks requiring a lot of thinking.
- Loses things.
- Is easily distracted.
- Is forgetful in daily activities.

Hyperactive-impulsive presentation:

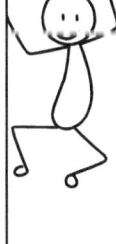

- Fidgets with hands or feet or squirms in chair.
- Has difficulty remaining seated.
- Runs about or climbs excessively in children; extreme restlessness in adults.
- Difficulty engaging in activities quietly.
- Acts as if driven by a motor; adults will often feel inside like they were driven by a motor.
- Talks excessively.
- Blurts out answers before questions have been completed.
- Difficulty waiting or taking turns.
- Interrupts or intrudes upon others.

Combined inattentive & hyperactive-impulsive presentation:

- Has symptoms from both of the above presentations

ADHD Diagnosis in Children

To diagnose a child with ADHD, a healthcare provider will complete the following steps:

- Interview parents or guardians, school staff, and mental health practitioners involved with the child about their academic or behavioral problems (such as struggles with grades or maintaining friendships)
- Assess the child's symptoms using tools such as behavior rating scales or checklists to ensure DSM-5 criteria for an ADHD diagnosis are met
- Complete a physical exam and order laboratory or other tests to rule out other conditions with similar symptoms, such as a seizure disorder, thyroid disorder, sleep disorders, or lead poisoning
- Run additional screening tests for co-occurring or other mental health conditions, including depression, anxiety, learning and language disorders, autism spectrum disorder, oppositional defiant disorder, conduct disorder, and tic disorders4
- Depending on the child's symptoms, you may also need a referral to meet with a pediatric specialist for additional screenings for conditions like developmental disorders or learning disabilities.

Impulsive children with ADHD may have trouble controlling their urges. They might not be able to stop and think before acting, which can lead to problems. When they do something impulsive, they may not understand why people get upset. They might think it's unfair because they didn't mean to be bad.

If left unchecked, impulsiveness can affect a child's behavior, schoolwork, self-esteem, and friendships. They might have trouble getting along with others and staying focused. Impulsive kids might also accidentally bother other children, making them seem bossy or mean.

It's important to remember that these kids don't always mean to be impulsive. Sometimes, they can't help it.

Ruling Out Other Possibilities

ADHD isn't always the only explanation for certain symptoms. Other conditions, like learning disabilities, autism, anxiety, depression, or even sleep or diet problems, can sometimes look like ADHD. It's important to check for these other possibilities first.

Building a Complete Picture

To diagnose ADHD, a doctor or therapist will ask about the child's behavior at home, school, and other places. Some pediatricians can do this, but often they'll refer families to a specialist who knows a lot about childhood conditions like ADHD.

Teachers as Partners

Teachers often spot signs of ADHD in their students. It's helpful for them to let the child's family know about their observations. This information can help the family and doctor figure out if the child has ADHD. The doctor might even give the teacher special forms to fill out about the child's behavior at school.

Collaboration is Key

Parents, teachers, and healthcare professionals can work together to make sure children with possible ADHD get the right evaluation and diagnosis.

Myths about Attention Deficit Disorder	
MYTH	**FACT**
All children with ADD/ADHD are hyperactive.	Some children with ADD/ADHD are hyperactive, but many others with attention problems are not. Children with ADD/ADHD, who are inattentive, but not overly active, may appear to be spacey and uninterested.
Children with ADD/ADHD never pay attention.	Children with ADD/ADHD are often able to concentrate on activities they enjoy. But no matter how hard they try, they have trouble maintaining focus when the task at hand appears to be boring or repetitive.
Children with ADD/ADHD choose to be difficult and could behave better if they wanted to.	Children with ADD/ADHD may do their best to be good, but still be unable to sit still, stay quiet, or pay attention. They may appear defiant, but that doesn't mean they're acting out on purpose.

Myths about Attention Deficit Disorder

MYTH	FACT
ADHD is just a phase children will grow out of.	ADHD is a neurodevelopmental disorder that persists throughout a person's life, although symptoms may change over time.
ADHD is caused by poor parenting or a lack of discipline.	ADHD is a biological disorder that has a strong genetic component. It's not caused by bad parenting or a child's willful behavior.
ADHD is a mental illness.	While ADHD can be considered a neurodevelopmental disorder, it's not a mental illness in the traditional sense. It doesn't involve severe emotional disturbances or hallucinations.
Children with ADHD are lazy or unmotivated.	Children with ADHD often struggle with focus, organization, and self-control, which can make it difficult for them to complete tasks. However, they are not lazy or unmotivated.
ADHD medication is a quick fix.	Medication can be a helpful tool for managing ADHD symptoms, but it's not a cure-all. It often works best when combined with other interventions, such as therapy and behavioral strategies.

CHAPTER 7
Autism

Scan QR code for more information on this chapter

Autism Spectrum Disorder

According to the CDC, autism spectrum disorders (ASDs) are a group of developmental disabilities that can cause significant social, communication and behavioral challenges (CDC 2008).

The DSM-5 TR identifies two major diagnosis criteria.

- The **first** is persistent deficits in social communication and social interaction across multiple contexts.
- The **second** is restricted, repetitive patterns of behavior, interest, or activities.

Symptoms must be present in early childhood and result in impairment in social, occupational or other area of function. ASD is defined by severity level. Severity level is defined by the amount of support the individual needs in social communication and restricted, repetitive behaviors. Level 1 requires support, level 2 requires substantial support and level 3 requires very substantial support (50).

According to the CDC, autism spectrum disorders (ASDs) are a group of developmental disabilities that can cause significant social, communication and behavioral challenges (CDC 2008).

The DSM-5 TR identifies two major diagnosis criteria.

- The **first** is persistent deficits in social communication and social interaction across multiple contexts.
- The **second** is restricted, repetitive patterns of behavior, interest, or activities.

Full-time childcare providers have a unique opportunity to recognize signs of autism spectrum disorder in children as they spend most of the child's waking hours with them. They can serve as a valuable resource for parents and healthcare providers, potentially aiding in the early detection of autism spectrum disorder through their presence and attentiveness. If caregivers suspect a child may be on the autism spectrum, sharing their concerns with parents can assist in timely detection and intervention.

The Role of Early Care and Education Providers

While specialists are responsible for diagnosing and providing targeted interventions for young children with ASD, early childhood providers can actively support children with autism and other developmental disabilities. By implementing developmentally appropriate practices, monitoring developmental milestones, engaging with parents, and staying informed about community resources, early care and education providers can significantly impact the lives of young children with ASD and their families.

Symptoms of Autism (ASD)

Symptoms must be present in early childhood and result in impairment in social, occupational or other area of function. ASD is defined by severity level. Severity level is defined by the amount of support the individual needs in social communication and restricted, repetitive behaviors. Level 1 requires support, level 2 requires substantial support and level 3 requires very substantial support (50).

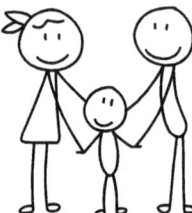

Level 1: Requires Support
Level 1 ASD describes people who do not need a lot of support. People with level 1 ASD may have a hard time communicating with neurotypical people, including their peers. For example, they may not say the right thing at the right time or be able to read social cues and body language.

A person labeled with ASD level 1 is usually able to communicate in full sentences most of the time, but may have trouble engaging in extended, back-and-forth communication with neurotypical people. They are likely to have social anxiety and may experience burnout from long term masking, or acting neurotypical.

They may also have trouble moving from one activity to another or trying new things. Additionally, they may have problems with organization and planning, and independence for them may differ from neurotypical expectations for people their age.

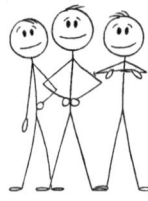

Level 2: Requires Substantial Support
People diagnosed with ASD level 2 have a harder time masking than those diagnosed with level 1 and may find it hard to communicate or socialize in ways that are accepted or understood by neurotypical society. Likewise, they will find it harder to change focus or shift from one activity to the next.

The DSM's level 2 expression of autism includes people who have very specific interests and who engage in repetitive behaviors that veer far from accepted, neurotypical behaviors or that appear in spaces neurotypical people view as incongruous.

For example, an autistic child or adult may pace back and forth during a class or meeting, or say the same thing over and over again. These behaviors are types of stimming, self-stimulation, that autistic people use to regulate themselves internally. Neurotypical people stim as well by humming, tapping their feet or fingers, dancing, etc.

One reason autistic people stim more is because most of our society was not built with neurodivergent people in mind. Hence, the regulation that is typically covered by societal infrastructure for neurotypical people has to be handled by autistic individuals and their loved ones. Autistic people who express level 2 and 3 traits have a larger burden of self-regulation.

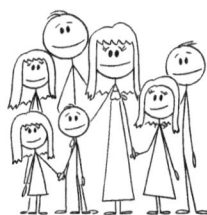

Level 3: Requires Very Substantial Support
People with level 3 diagnoses need the most support and are subsequently at very high risk for neglect, abuse, and discrimination. People in this category will have many of the same traits as those with levels 1 and 2 diagnoses, but are entirely unable to mask and have very high burdens of self-regulation.

Problems expressing themselves accurately both verbally and with body language or facial expressions can make it very hard to complete daily living tasks, interact socially, and deal with a change in focus or location. Some of these difficulties can be assuaged with early access to augmentative and alternative communication (AAC) devices, as communication is a human right everyone should have access to even if they do not speak. Engaging in repetitive behaviors is another trait of level 3 ASD.

A person with an ASD level 3 diagnosis is more likely to have communication differences and may rarely initiate interactions, especially with neurotypical people. When they do, they are likely to be perceived as awkward.3 They may be more comfortable with or prefer parallel play instead of interactive hangouts, or might prefer to interact with other based upon scripts.

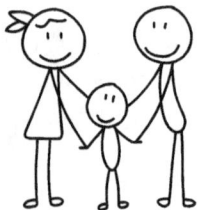
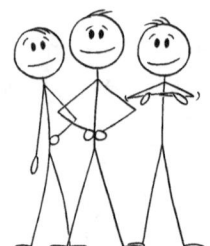
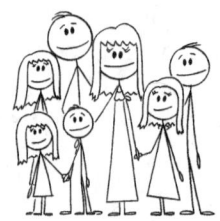

Level 1:
Requiring Support

Level 2:
Requiring Substantial Support

Level 3:
Requiring Very Substantial Support

- Lowest Level and highest functioning
- Difficulty initiating social interactions
- Decreasing interest in social interactions
- Struggling with switching between activities
- Organizing and planning problems

- Social impairments even with support
- Problems with verbal and nonverbal communication
- Struggling coping with change
- Changing focus or activities can cause distress
- Frequently appearing restrictive or repetitive behavior

- Severe problems with verbal and nonverbal communication
- Frequently appearing restrictive or repetitive behaviors that interfere with daily functioning in all aspects of life
- Changing focus or activities cause serve stress.
- Extreme difficulty coping with change
- Rarely speaking logically and with few words

Many may or may not know of Dr. Temple Grandin, Ph.D.; she is well known in different circles for vastly different reasons. In the educational/autistic population she is known for over coming her challenges with Autism during a time that not much was known about the disorder; she also has a Ph.D. in animal husbandry and teaches at Colorado State University.

In the book *The Way I See It*, Temple Grandin explains that individuals with autism have different ways of thinking thus learning. The different types outlined in her book are:

Visual thinkers- love art and building blocks. They tend to take longer responding verbally. These children think in realistic pictures, they tend to produce beautiful drawings.

Music/Math thinkers- patterns verses pictures dominate the thinking processes. If you think about it music and math are made of patterns. Good at music and math.

Verbal thinkers- love lists and numbers. These children tend to memorize events in history, routes. These children may learn different languages easily. The thinking patterns of these children are different than "Typical" people, thus often too much emphasis is placed on what they can't do verses what they can do. (pg19, Gradin)

Expecting a child with autism to learn the conventional curriculum and teaching methods that have worked for neuro-typical children is to set everyone up for failure. Good teachers understand that for a child to learn the teaching style must match the students learning style.

A few things to remember about a student with autism:

- Learning rules is easy but learning flexibility in thinking is difficult and must be taught.
- Children on the spectrum have areas of strengths and an area of deficits
- There are different functioning levels of person's with Autism.
- They are not all the same.

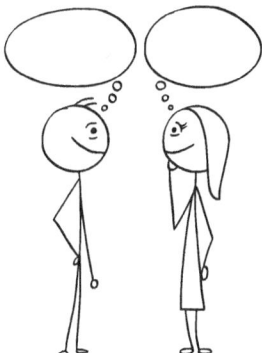

Social communication and interaction skills can be challenging for people with ASD.

Examples of social communication and social interaction characteristics related to ASD can include
- Avoids or does not keep eye contact
- Does not respond to name by 9 months of age
- Does not show facial expressions like happy, sad, angry, and surprised by 9 months of age
- Does not play simple interactive games like pat-a-cake by 12 months of age
- Uses few or no gestures by 12 months of age (for example, does not wave goodbye)
- Does not share interests with others by 15 months of age (for example, shows you an object that they like)
- Does not point to show you something interesting by 18 months of age
- Does not notice when others are hurt or upset by 24 months of age
- Does not notice other children and join them in play by 36 months of age
- Does not pretend to be something else, like a teacher or superhero, during play by 48 months of age
- Does not sing, dance, or act for you by 60 months of age

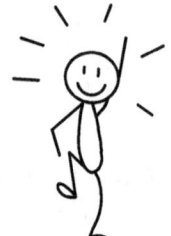 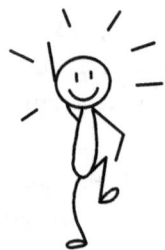 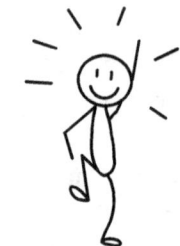

People with ASD have behaviors or interests that can seem unusual. These behaviors or interests set ASD apart from conditions defined by problems with social communication and interaction only.

Examples of restricted or repetitive behaviors and interests related to ASD can include:

- Arranges toys or objects in a specific order and becomes upset when the order is disrupted
- Repeats words or phrases repeatedly, known as echolalia
- Engages in repetitive play patterns with toys
- Shows a strong focus on specific parts of objects, such as wheels
- Reacts strongly to minor changes
- Demonstrates obsessive interests
- Requires adherence to particular routines
- Engages in hand flapping, body rocking, or spinning in circles
- Exhibits unusual responses to sensory stimuli, including sounds, smells, tastes, appearances, or textures

Individuals with ASD often exhibit other associated traits, such as:

- Delayed language abilities
- Delayed motor skills
- Delayed cognitive or learning capabilitie
- Hyperactive, impulsive, or inattentive conduct
- Epilepsy or seizure conditions
- Unconventional eating and sleeping patterns
- Gastrointestinal problems (e.g., constipation)
- Unusual emotional responses or moods
- Anxiety, stress, or heightened worry
- Absence of fear or heightened fear levels

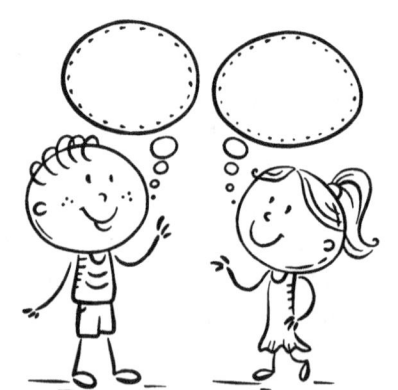

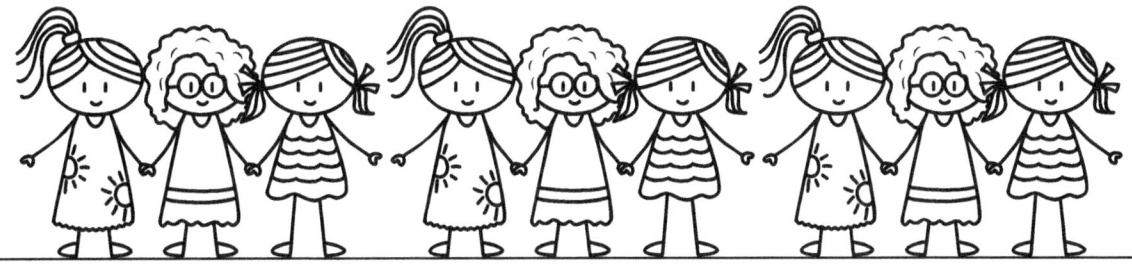

Understanding Autism in Girls

It's becoming increasingly clear that girls with autism spectrum disorder (ASD) often present differently than boys. While the current diagnosis ratio is skewed towards boys, there's growing evidence suggesting that many girls with autism may be going undiagnosed.

One reason for this is that girls with autism often exhibit behaviors that are more "typical" for their gender. They may be better at masking or camouflaging their autistic traits, meaning they consciously or unconsciously hide behaviors that might be seen as "different." This can make it harder to identify autism in girls, as their symptoms may not be as immediately obvious.

Masking can also have a negative impact on girls' mental health. It can lead to feelings of exhaustion, stress, and depression. Additionally, masking can delay diagnosis, which means girls may not receive the support they need.

Another factor contributing to the underdiagnosis of autism in girls is that they may not exhibit the same stereotypical behaviors as boys. For example, girls might not line up toys or flap their hands, but they may have repetitive behaviors like rereading books or watching the same show over and over. These behaviors may be seen as normal or "typical" for girls, making it harder to recognize them as signs of autism.

Overall, it's important to be aware of the unique ways that girls with autism may present. By understanding these differences, we can help ensure that more girls receive the early diagnosis and support they need to thrive.

Individuals with ASD commonly experience various mental health conditions:

- ADHD affects 50-70% of the ASD population.
- Depression affects 26% of the ASD population compared to 10% of the general population.
- Anxiety affects 30% of the ASD population compared to 10% of the general population.
- Bipolar Disorder affects 11% of the ASD population compared to 2% of the general population.
- Schizophrenia affects 7% of the ASD population compared to 0.5% of the general population.
- The most commonly diagnosed comorbidities are ADHD, anxiety, and depression.

85% of children with autism also have a comorbid psychiatric diagnosis, with 35% receiving psychotropic medication as treatment (Bennett, 2022).

Around 50% to 80% of children with autism experience sleep disorders, including difficulty falling asleep, frequent waking, and early rising.

Gastrointestinal (GI) disorders are prevalent among individuals with ASD, affecting 46% to 84% of the population. Common GI symptoms in the ASD population include food intolerance, nausea, vomiting, abdominal pain, constipation, diarrhea, gastroesophageal reflux, ulcers, colitis, and failure to thrive.

Caring for Children with ASD

Because children on the autism spectrum may behave and respond differently than their peers, it's important for childcare providers to have a basic understanding of the appropriate care methods.

Provide Consistency –One of the common difficulties faced by children on the spectrum is trouble adapting lessons learned in one setting to another. This means a child who uses sign language to communicate at home may not necessarily communicate in this manner in a childcare setting, for instance. Childcare providers who are committed to providing some consistency for the children under their care who have ASD should work closely with parents to encourage interaction and the use of acquired skills in a variety of settings.

Build a Routine –Childcare in a group setting is often built around a daily schedule, but it becomes especially important to adhere to this schedule as closely as possible when there's a child with ADS in the group. These children respond best and thrive when their routine is highly structured and dependable. Minimizing schedule disruptions and preparing children in advance for a significant change can help to reduce the likelihood of unfavorable reactions.

Offer Direct Praise –Most children do well when they're actively praised, but children on the spectrum need very specific praise in order to reinforce good behavior. Childcare providers who "catch" a child on the spectrum behaving well should not only praise the child, but also let them know why they're receiving the positive attention.

Be Aware of Sensory Processing Differences –Children on the autism spectrum may be highly sensitive to smell, light, sound, taste and touch, or they may be markedly less sensitive to everyday stimuli than their peers. For children whose ASD is accompanied by hypersensitivity, over-stimulation can elicit outbursts or disruptive behavior. Caregivers should make a point of paying attention to the way children on the spectrum react to stimuli, and helping to minimize discomfort for those with hypersensitivities.

CHAPTER 8
Adverse Childhood Experiences

Scan QR code for more information on this chapter

Adverse Childhood Experiences (ACEs) are traumatic events that occur before the age of 18. These experiences can have a profound impact on a child's development and well-being.

Common ACEs include:
- Physical, sexual, and emotional abuse
- Neglect (emotional or physical)
- Witnessing domestic violence
- Living with a family member with substance abuse or mental health issues
- Sudden separation from a loved one
- Poverty
- Racism or discrimination
- Violence in the community
- Natural disasters

When the stress response is triggered repeatedly over a prolonged period of time it physically alters the brain, leaving certain parts rewired – adapted for surviving danger.

The amygdala of a child living with trauma is likely to be in overdrive, constantly signalling danger, releasing cortisol and priming them for fight, flight, freeze or fawn responses.

Research has shown a strong correlation between the number of ACEs a child experiences and their risk of developing various health problems later in life, such as:

- Heart disease
- Diabetes
- Obesity
- Depression
- Substance abuse
- Smoking
- Poor academic performance
- Early death

Repeated exposure to stress can physically alter the brain, leaving it primed for a constant state of alert. This can lead to feelings of fear, anxiety, and hypersensitivity to everyday stimuli. Children may also develop coping mechanisms like people-pleasing or excessive vigilance to maintain a sense of safety.

The amygdala, often referred to as the "fear center," plays a crucial role in stress responses. In children who have experienced trauma, the amygdala may be hyperactive, constantly signaling danger and releasing cortisol. This can lead to a heightened state of arousal, preparing the child for a fight, flight, freeze, or fawn response.

Trauma can also affect the prefrontal cortex, known as the "thinking center." This part of the brain is responsible for cognitive functions like concentration, decision-making, and processing new information. Trauma can disrupt these functions, making it more challenging for children to focus and learn.

The anterior cingulate cortex, or "emotional regulation center," may also be impacted by trauma. This can lead to difficulties in managing strong emotions and maintaining emotional balance.

Additionally, trauma can affect the hippocampus, a brain region involved in memory formation and retrieval. Traumatic memories may be stored in a way that makes them seem more current than past events, causing children to experience flashbacks or triggers. These triggers can be anything from sounds, smells, or environments to images, movements, or touch.

Children who experience traumatic events may feel helpless and vulnerable, especially if they cannot rely on adults for protection. This can lead to them reenacting the event in pretend play or having nightmares about it. This can lead to behavioral changes, such as:

- **Emotional distress:** Clinginess, temper tantrums, nightmares
- **Social withdrawal:** Avoiding social interactions
- **Difficulty focusing:** Struggling to concentrate or complete tasks
- **Aggressive behavior:** Acting out towards others

These children may also find it challenging to interact positively with teachers and family members.

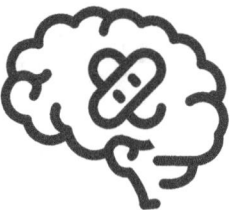

> Persistent exposure to traumatic events, such as community violence or domestic abuse, can lead to chronic stress in children and youth. This ongoing stress can disrupt brain development and hinder social and emotional growth. Known as toxic stress, this condition can impact a child's behavior at home and school, potentially shaping their development into adulthood.

Trauma

Trauma, literally meaning a wound, shock, or injury, can also refer to emotional distress caused by an overwhelming event. This event, whether singular or recurring, is perceived as harmful or life-threatening to oneself or loved ones. Individual reactions to trauma vary; what one person finds traumatic may not affect another. Studies indicate that nearly one-quarter of American children experience a traumatic event before their fourth birthday.

The Different Forms of Trauma
Trauma manifests in various ways, each impacting mental well-being differently.

Acute trauma:
- Involves intense distress immediately following a brief, one-time event.
- This reaction is short-lived and often resolves on its own or with counseling.
- Examples include car accidents, physical or sexual assaults, sudden loss of a loved one, or medical emergencies.

Chronic trauma:
- Results from prolonged or repetitive events, causing lasting harm.
- Stemming from ongoing bullying, neglect, emotional, physical, or sexual abuse, and domestic violence.
- Due to its persistent nature, chronic trauma can have severe mental health repercussions

Complex trauma:
- Arises from enduring multiple or repeated traumatic experiences with no means of escape, such as repeated childhood abuse.
- The feeling of being trapped is a key aspect of this experience.
- Like other types of trauma, it can erode a sense of safety in the world and lead to hypervigilance.

Secondary or vicarious trauma:
- Develops from exposure to the suffering of others, particularly affecting professionals like physicians, first responders, and law enforcement.
- Over time, individuals in these roles are at risk for compassion fatigue, leading them to emotionally disengage to protect themselves from distress

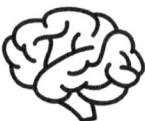

Children who have or are currently experiencing adverse childhood experiences need security and understanding. Provide support and resources to the primary caregivers and recommend counseling for the child.

If you suspect a child is currently being abused, you are required to report to the local authorities.

CHAPTER 9
Childhood Depression, Anxiety and Behavior

Scan QR code for more information on this chapter

Depression and Anxiety

Childhood depression, a mood disorder characterized by persistent sadness, irritability, or hopelessness, can significantly impact a child's life. Unlike typical mood swings, depression in children lasts for more than two weeks. It can interfere with sleep, appetite, relationships, and enjoyment of activities. In severe cases, it may even lead to suicidal thoughts.

Approximately 3% of children and adolescents aged 3 to 17 experience depression, with higher rates among teenagers. Major depression affects about one in five teenagers, but many cases remain undiagnosed. Children and adolescents with chronic health conditions such as diabetes, epilepsy, chronic pain, and asthma may be at a higher risk of depression.

Clinically significant depression can appear in children as young as three years old. There is a lack of data on the prevalence of depression in preschool-aged children. Current studies indicate that both boys and girls are affected to the same extent.

What Causes Childhood Depression?

The exact causes of depression in children and adolescents remain unclear, but it's believed to be influenced by both genetics and environmental factors. Several factors may contribute to childhood depression, including:

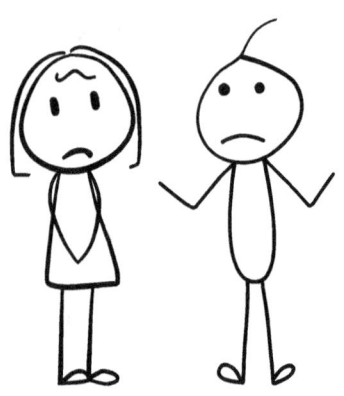

- **Genetics and family history:** A family history of depression can increase the risk.

- **Physical health:** Illnesses or injuries can contribute to depressive symptoms.

- **Stressful life events:** Divorce, moving, or the loss of a loved one can be triggers.

- **Bullying and trauma:** Negative experiences can impact mental health.

Risk Factors for Childhood Depression

- **Family history:** A close relative with depression.

- **Personal history:** Prior depression, anxiety, gender identity issues, ADHD, or conduct problems.

- **Adverse childhood experiences:** Trauma or neglect.

- **Bullying:** Negative social experiences.

- **Family conflicts:** Stressful home environment.

- **Loss:** The death of a loved one or relationship difficulties

- **Medical factors:** Low birth weight, brain injury, or chronic illnesses.

- **Social challenges:** Friendship problems.

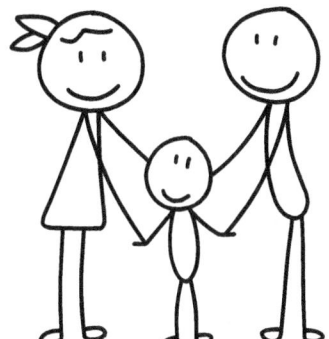

> While genetics may contribute to a child's susceptibility to depression, in preschool-aged children, depression predominantly arises from environmental factors leading to psychosocial stress. These issues may stem from an unfavorable home environment, a caregiver dealing with depression or a severe illness, challenging peer interactions, and stressful life events like the loss of a parent or separation from a significant individual in the child's life.
>
> Typically, young children experiencing depression often show physical symptoms like frequent headaches or stomachaches, along with alterations in their sleep patterns, appetite, and social behavior. Sleep changes may involve difficulties falling asleep, staying asleep, or oversleeping. In preschoolers, appetite problems usually manifest as not eating enough rather than overeating. Additionally, their mood might be characterized by irritability rather than explicit sadness.

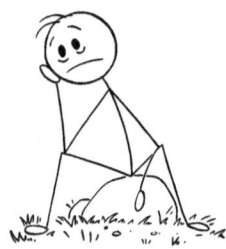

Signs and Symptoms of Depression in Preschoolers

If you notice any of the following changes in your child that persist for more than two weeks, they might be experiencing depression:

Emotional Changes:
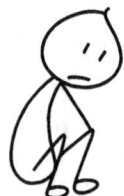
- Persistent sadness or unhappiness.
- Frequent fear or worry.
- Easy irritability or anger.
- Frustration and avoidance of challenges.
- Excessive guilt or worry about mistakes.

Behavioral Changes:
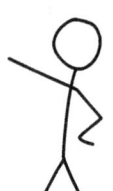
- Separation anxiety.
- Defiance or frequent tantrums.
- Aggression, self-harm, or property damage.
- Negative self-talk (e.g., "I'm not good at anything").
- Excessive blame or apologies.
- Difficulty speaking and emotional outbursts.
- Easy giving up and negative statements.

Preschool Behavior:
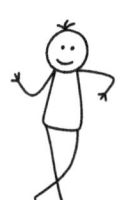
- Timidity or withdrawal.
- Disengagement from preschool activities.
- Social isolation.
- Difficulty interacting with peers.
- Increased challenging behaviors (e.g., tantrums, aggression).

Changes in Interests and Activities:

- Loss of interest in previously enjoyed activities.
- Preference for violent or negative themes.
- Social withdrawal.
- Concentration and memory problems.

Physical Changes:
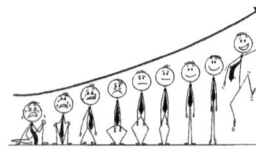
- Low energy levels.
- Sleep disturbances, including nightmares.
- Significant weight gain or loss.
- Appetite changes (e.g., overeating or refusing food).
- Persistent unexplained physical symptoms (e.g., stomach pain, headaches).

Anxiety

When a child's fears and worries persist beyond what is typical for their age or significantly interfere with daily life, they may be diagnosed with an anxiety disorder.

Examples of anxiety disorders include:

- **Separation anxiety:** Excessive fear of being away from parents or caregivers.

- **Phobias:** Intense fear of a specific object or situation (e.g., animals, heights, needles).

- **Social anxiety:** Fear of social situations and interactions.

- **Generalized anxiety disorder:** Excessive worry about various future events.

- **Panic disorder:** Sudden, intense fear attacks accompanied by physical symptoms (e.g., rapid heartbeat, shortness of breath).

Anxiety can manifest as fear or worry, but it can also lead to irritability and anger. Other symptoms may include sleep disturbances, fatigue, headaches, and stomachaches. Some anxious children may hide their worries, making it difficult to recognize the disorder.

Around 1 in 5 children may experience anxiety disorders, as recognized by healthcare providers. Childhood anxiety disorders are distinct from normal fear or anxiety due to their heightened avoidance behaviors, intense emotional responses, or prolonged durations.

Children with anxiety disorders may exhibit emotional outbursts such as crying or tantrums, along with frequent avoidance tactics like trying to escape, hide, or remain vigilant for potential threats. Furthermore, these children may also present physical symptoms like stomachaches, headaches, nausea, vomiting, shortness of breath, or sleep disturbances.

Separation Anxiety Disorder

Separation anxiety is a common developmental phase that typically begins around 8-12 months. While normal separation anxiety involves fear of strangers and discomfort when caregivers are absent, separation anxiety disorder is more severe and persists beyond the usual developmental period. Children with this disorder may experience intense distress, difficulty with separations, and avoidance of school or unfamiliar settings. If your child exhibits excessive separation anxiety compared to their peers or shows no improvement over time, consult with their healthcare provider.

Specific Phobias: A certain degree of fear is normal in children. However, specific phobias are extreme, disproportionate fears of specific objects or situations. For example, a child might have an intense fear of storms, clowns, or other things.

Specific Phobias: A certain degree of fear is normal in children. However, specific phobias are extreme, disproportionate fears of specific objects or situations. For example, a child might have an intense fear of storms, clowns, or other things.

- **Social Anxiety Disorder:** This disorder involves an overwhelming fear of social judgment or rejection. Children with social anxiety may avoid public speaking, performances, or social interactions. They might struggle to speak to new people or feel uncomfortable in familiar settings.

- **Generalized Anxiety Disorder:** Excessive worry and fear about everyday life characterize generalized anxiety disorder. Children with this condition may often worry about the future and experience a range of concerns that can change over time.

- **Panic Disorder:** Panic disorder involves sudden, intense fear attacks accompanied by physical symptoms like rapid heartbeat, dizziness, shortness of breath, or a sense of impending doom. These attacks can occur without warning and typically last for minutes to hours.

Behavior

Behavior is defined as the way in which one acts or conducts oneself. Behavior is a form of communication. Behavior in of itself can be good or bad.

Behavior is a form of communication. While it can be positive or negative, challenging behaviors often require deeper investigation to understand the underlying causes.

Identifying the Root Cause:
- **Context**: Consider the location, environment, and recent changes.
- **Triggers**: Determine what preceded the behavior (people, activities, sensory changes).
- **Reactions**: Observe the child's reaction and any responses from others.
- **Duration**: Note the length of the behavior.
- **Resolution**: Understand how the behavior ended.

Beyond Behavior:
- **Age and development**: Consider the child's developmental stage and abilities.
- **Cognitive and language skills**: Assess their understanding and communication abilities.
- **Emotional literacy:** Evaluate their ability to identify and express their own emotions, as well as those of others.

By analyzing these components, we can gain a better understanding of challenging behaviors and develop effective strategies for addressing them.

There are multiple components that must be looked at when addressing behaviors.

- **First, where did the behavior change?**
    - What location?
    - What is the environment of that location?
    - Is this a new or unfamiliar environment?

- **Second, what happened just before the behavior was noticed?**
    - What changed?
    - Who was in the room?
    - Who left the room?
    - Was there a change of activities?
    - Was there any change in the environment such as smells or lighting?

- **Third, who was with the child or next to the child?**

- **Fourth, What reaction did the child receive when the behavior began?**

- **Fifth, how long did the behavior last? Lastly, how did the behavior stop?**

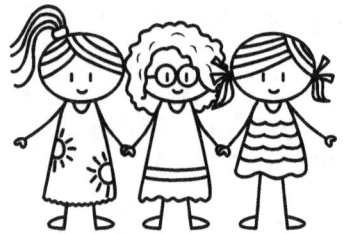

In addition to the above components, you must also consider the child's age and developmental ability. Specifically, it is important to understand the child's cognitive and language ability as well as their emotional literacy. Emotional literacy is a child's ability to label and talk about their own emotions or feelings, as well as the feelings and emotions of others.

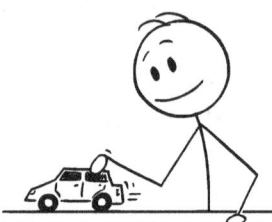

It is common to interpret a child throwing toys at you as a sign of anger due to their outward display of emotion. However, the child might actually be overstimulated and in a fight-or-flight response. The act of throwing toys could be their way of self-protection. The child may also be excessively tired and struggling to communicate their feelings verbally. The toy-throwing behavior could be a response to emotions that the child may find challenging to comprehend or express in a suitable manner.

When children feel upset or threatened, their ability to process information and express emotions can be impaired. This state, often referred to as "fight or flight," is an automatic physiological response to perceived stress or danger. Activated by the sympathetic nervous system, this response prepares the body for action by triggering a surge of adrenaline.

The **"fight" response** involves aggression or confrontation, while the **"flight" response** urges escape. The **"freeze" response**, characterized by immobility, can also occur.

Fight Mode: When your body perceives a threat it believes it can overcome, it enters "fight mode." The brain signals the body to prepare for physical confrontation.

Signs of fight mode include:
- Tight jaw or clenched teeth
- Urge to punch or hit
- Intense anger
- Stomping or kicking
- Crying out of anger
- Stomach discomfort or tension
- Aggressive behavior towards the perceived threat

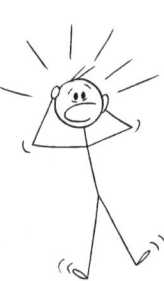

Flight mode is a physiological response triggered by the body when it perceives a threat that it cannot overcome. In this state, the body's instinct is to escape the danger.

Signs of flight mode may include:
- Rapid heartbeat
- Increased breathing rate
- Sweating
- Feeling lightheaded or dizzy
- Nausea
- Urge to run away or hide

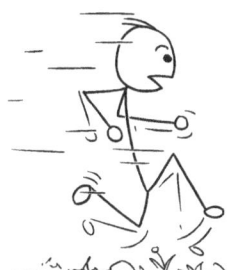

Essentially, the body prepares itself for physical exertion to flee from the perceived threat.

Freeze Mode: When your body perceives a threat it cannot overcome, it enters "freeze mode."

This response involves feeling paralyzed or unable to act.

Signs of freeze mode include:
- **Emotional distress:** Sense of dread, fear
- **Physical sensations:** Pale skin, stiffness, heaviness, coldness, numbness
- **Breathing patterns:** Holding breath, rapid or slowed heartbeat
- **Mental states:** Shutting down, feeling unable to move, escaping into thoughts
- **Vocalizations:** Whining, daydreaming

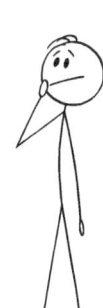

Note: These are common signs, but individual responses may vary.

When a child is in fight, flight, or freeze mode, focus on their breathing. Regulated breathing can help activate the prefrontal cortex, or "upstairs brain."

Avoid saying "calm down." Instead, use simple phrases like **"let's breathe"** or **"in through the nose, out through the mouth."** Reasoning or lecturing won't be effective at this stage.

Crossing midline exercises can help rebalance brain hemispheres and activate the prefrontal cortex.

Once breathing is regulated, try other calming techniques:
- Squeezing a stress ball
- Spending time in a sensory room or calm-down area
- Blowing bubbles
- Coloring
- Yoga poses
- Chewing bubble gum
- Sensory activities (especially heavy work)
- Using a calm-down bottle

Experiment to find the most effective techniques for your child.

Emotional literacy is a cornerstone of social-emotional development. It enables children to understand their own emotions and empathize with others. By labeling and discussing their feelings, children can better regulate their emotions and solve problems. These skills are crucial for success in preschool and beyond.

Children who are emotionally literate are more likely to:

- **Focus on tasks:** Stay engaged in classroom activities.
- **Manage emotions:** Avoid frustration, tantrums, and impulsivity.

Behavioral Developmental Milestones

Behavioral development encompasses a child's emotional, social, and communication skills.

Here are some key milestones across different age groups:

Infancy (0-12 months):
- Social-emotional: Smiles, laughs, shows interest in others, displays separation anxiety.
- Communication: Cries, coos, babbles, responds to sounds.

Toddlerhood (1-3 years):
- Social-emotional: Plays alongside others, shows empathy, understands simple rules, exhibits temper tantrums.
- Communication: Says single words, combines words into phrases, follows simple instructions.

Preschool (3-5 years):
- Social-emotional: Shares toys, takes turns, expresses feelings, shows independence.
- Communication: Uses complete sentences, follows complex instructions, engages in pretend play.

Elementary School (6-12 years):
- Social-emotional: Forms friendships, understands social cues, manages emotions, develops a sense of self.

Communication: Speaks fluently, expresses opinions, participates in group discussions.
Remember, these are general milestones, and individual children may develop at different rates. If you have concerns about your child's behavior, consult with a healthcare professional.

CHAPTER 10
Sleep Disorders and Nutrition

Scan QR code for more information on this chapter

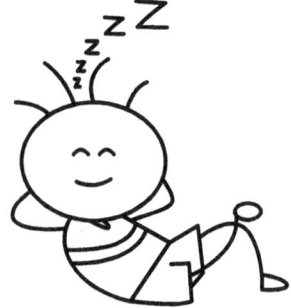

Sleep Disorders

Sleep is crucial for giving our body and brain the needed rest. It enables our body to rejuvenate the immune, nervous, skeletal, and muscular systems, which are essential for regulating mood, memory, and cognitive function. Sleep plays a vital role in every aspect of a child's growth. Insufficient restful sleep can affect a child's focus, emotional management, and learning abilities.

Over time, insufficient sleep can lead to various physical, emotional, and mental alterations in children, such as:
- Daytime sleepiness
- Changes in mood
- Difficulty regulating emotions
- Weakened immune system
- Impaired memory
- Reduced problem-solving abilities
- Decline in overall health
- Irritability in younger children is frequently an indication of inadequate sleep

> Researchers discovered that children who lacked sufficient sleep at the beginning of the study faced more mental health and behavioral difficulties compared to those who had adequate sleep. These challenges included impulsivity, stress, depression, anxiety, aggressive behavior, and cognitive issues. The children with insufficient sleep also showed decreased cognitive functions like decision-making, problem-solving, working memory, and learning.
>
> Children who had less than nine hours of sleep per night initially had reduced grey matter or smaller volume in specific brain areas responsible for attention, memory, and impulse control, in contrast to those with healthy sleep patterns.

Insufficient sleep refers to not getting enough rest, which can be influenced by various factors.

A child's sleep can be affected by their environment, such as inadequate bedding or discomfort due to sensory issues. The room setup may not be conducive to sleep, with too many toys or unfavorable colors or temperatures. Feeling unsafe or disturbances like noise can also disrupt a child's sleep. Additionally, having a television on or using electronic devices at bedtime has been linked to shorter sleep duration, lower sleep quality, and increased daytime drowsiness based on consistent research findings.

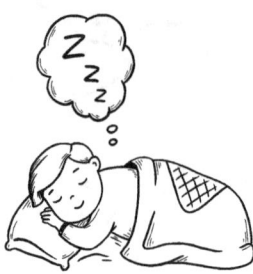

The American Academy of Pediatrics estimates that 25-50% of children experience sleep problems.

These disorders fall into two main categories: dyssomnia and parasomnia.
Dyssomnia refers to difficulties falling asleep or staying asleep.

Parasomnia involves abnormal behaviors during sleep, such as sleep terrors or sleepwalking.

Obstructive sleep apnea (OSA) is a serious medical condition that can affect children. During sleep, OSA causes partial or complete blockage of the upper airway, leading to disrupted breathing. This can occur multiple times per night.

Symptoms of pediatric OSA may include:

- Snoring
- Pauses in breathing
- Restless sleep
- Snorting, coughing, or choking
- Mouth breathing
- Nighttime sweating
- Bed-wetting
- Sleep terrors

The child' primary physician should be informed if a child presents with the above symptoms.

How much sleep do children need?
Time listed includes naps

- Newborn (birth to 3 months): 14 to 17 hours

- Infant (4 to 11 months): 12 to 16 hours

- Toddler (1 to 2 years): 11 to 14 hours

- Preschool/Kindergarten (3 to 5 years): 10 to 13 hours

Keep in mind, the number of hours listed above is for actual time asleep. When establishing a bedtime routine, keep in mind how long the process takes. Allow time for the child to wind down, bath time, brushing teeth and for a bed time story. If a child needs ten hours of sleep at night and must be up at 6:30 am, the child needs to be asleep by 8:30 pm. The bedtime routine should start no later than 8:00 pm.

Nutrition

Nutrition significantly influences the mental, social, physical, and behavioral growth of toddlers. Nowadays, children often lack a balance of nutrients, consuming excessive fats, sugars, and salt while not getting enough proteins, vitamins, and minerals. This dietary imbalance can have both immediate and long-lasting negative impacts on health, including stunted growth, obesity, mood fluctuations, decreased focus, heightened tantrums, and reduced mental and physical agility.

During toddlerhood, the brain undergoes rapid development, enhancing learning abilities and cognitive skills such as working memory and attention. Essential nutrients like choline, folic acid, iron, zinc, copper, iodine, selenium, vitamin A, and specific fats like gangliosides, sphingolipids, and docosahexaenoic acid are crucial for this process. Inadequate intake of these nutrients can hinder your toddler's brain development. Monitoring a child's mental developmental milestones is vital for evaluating brain growth.

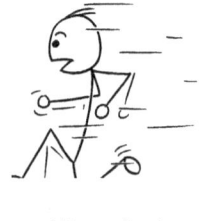

If your toddler displays signs such as excessive running around the house, destructive behavior, difficulty sleeping at night or focusing during the day, it could be linked to a nutritional deficiency. Additionally, they might exhibit visual and muscular coordination issues and struggle with basic problem-solving and decision-making.

Carbohydrates serve as the main energy source for the body, fueling physical activities and brain functions. The quality and quantity of carbohydrates eaten greatly affect a child's well-being. Consuming highly processed and refined carbohydrates like sugary snacks, sweetened drinks, and white bread can cause sudden spikes and drops in blood sugar levels. This fluctuation may lead to mood swings, tiredness, and concentration issues, ultimately affecting a child's learning and behavior. Sugar is often a major factor in mood swings and behavioral challenges.

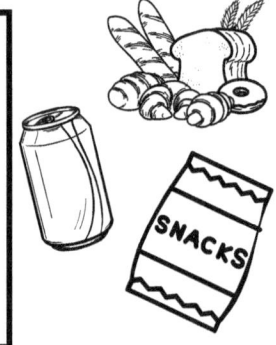

Health Impacts of Poor Diet and Hydration
- Poor diet and hydration can cause constipation, poor appetite, and stomach pain.
- Drinking enough water is crucial for circulation, metabolism, temperature regulation, and waste removal.
- Even mild dehydration can lead to headaches, irritability, reduced physical performance, and cognitive issues.

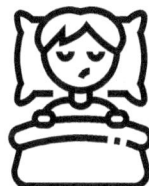

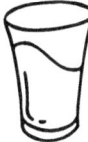

Nutritionist report on hydration for kids
- Water should be the main source of hydration for kids over 1 year old.
- Toddlers (ages 1-3) should drink 2-4 cups (16-32 ounces) of water daily.
- Children ages 4-5 should drink five cups of water per day.

Health Impacts of Poor Diet and Hydration
- Poor diet and hydration can lead to constipation, poor appetite, and stomach pain.
- Constipation may result in negative behaviors.
- Adequate water intake is crucial for circulation, metabolism, temperature regulation, and waste removal.
- Even mild dehydration can cause headaches, irritability, reduced physical performance, and cognitive issues.

The popularity of ultra-processed foods stems from their convenience and long shelf life, fitting well into our fast-paced modern lifestyles. Yet, regular consumption of these foods can have serious health consequences.

High intake of ultra-processed foods has been associated with health issues like obesity, heart disease, diabetes, and some types of cancer. Typically high in calories, sugars, unhealthy fats, and sodium, these foods lack essential nutrients such as fiber, vitamins, and minerals.

For a healthier lifestyle, experts often suggest prioritizing whole, minimally processed foods. Incorporating fresh fruits and vegetables, whole grains, lean proteins, and healthy fats from sources like nuts and avocados can provide the necessary nutrients for maintaining good health. Cooking meals at home with these ingredients can be a fulfilling way to ensure a nutritious and delicious diet.

Furthermore, paying attention to food labels and understanding ingredients can lead to better dietary decisions. Opt for products with fewer and recognizable ingredients, and try to reduce consumption of items with long lists of additives and preservatives.

By making mindful adjustments to our eating patterns, we can significantly enhance our overall well-being and contribute to a healthier future.

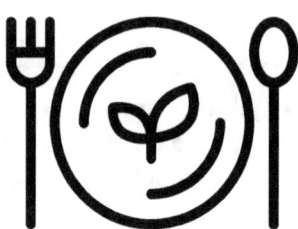

The Academy of Nutrition and Dietetics ranks processed foods from minimally to mostly or ultra-processed:

Ranking foods from minimally to ultra-processed
- **Minimally processed:** fresh blueberries, cut vegetables, roasted nuts.
- **Peak-processed:** canned tomatoes, tuna, frozen fruits/vegetables.
- **Added ingredients**: jarred pasta sauce, salad dressing, yogurt, cake mixes.
- Ready-to-eat: crackers, chips, deli meat.
- **Ultra-processed:** sweetened cereals, soda, energy drinks, flavored crackers, chicken nuggets, hot dogs.

Healthy diet considerations
- Minimally processed foods like low-fat milk, whole-grain bread, and precut vegetables are beneficial.
- Fortified dairy and plant-based milks, and breakfast cereals with added fiber, enhance nutrition.
- Canned fruits in water or natural juice are good alternatives when fresh fruit is unavailable.

Impact of High-Sugar Diet on Health
- Contributes to leptin resistance, affecting energy regulation and hunger.
- Linked to insulin resistance, weight gain, and type 2 diabetes.
- Alters hormones related to appetite, increasing ghrelin (hunger hormone) and lowering peptide2 (appetite-suppressing hormone).

Addictive Nature of Sugar
- Stimulates the brain's reward system (limbic system), leading to repeated consumption.

Impact on Children's Health
- Increases risk of tooth decay, a major reason for child hospital admissions.
- Poor oral hygiene from high sugar intake affects both milk teeth and future adult teeth.

Nutritional Deficiencies
- Children consuming high-sugar diets often lack essential nutrients like iron, calcium, and vitamins.
- Nutritional deficiencies during growth can impact health later in life.

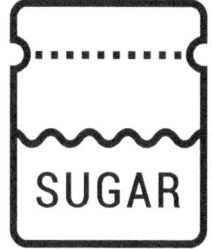

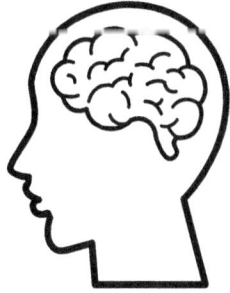

Brain Development and Sugar Consumption
- Research indicates that excessive sugar intake can impact brain development, as the brain relies on glucose for cognitive functions like thinking, learning, and memory.
- Consuming too much sugar has been associated with a higher risk of depression and anxiety, based on a study of over 23,000 individuals.
- The relationship between sugar consumption and mood disorders is still not fully understood.
- Sleep Quality and Sugar Intake
- A diet high in sugar can result in poor quality sleep, affecting a child's cognitive abilities.
- Quality sleep is crucial for children's development, influencing attention, memory, and self-control.
- Excessive sugar consumption in children can disrupt sleep patterns, negatively affecting their learning and behavior in school.

Ensuring adequate intake of these vitamins is crucial for a child's overall health and well-being. A balanced diet rich in whole foods, along with potential supplementation as recommended by a healthcare professional, can help meet these nutritional needs.

These essential nutrients support various bodily functions, including:

Vitamin	Benefits	Food Source
Vitamin A	Eye health, immune function, cell growth	Carrots, sweet potatoes, spinach, fortified milk, eggs
Vitamin B12	Brain and nerve function, red blood cell production	Meat, poultry, fish, eggs, fortified cereals
Vitamin C	Immune function, iron absorption, collagen production	Citrus fruits, strawberries, tomatoes, broccoli
Vitamin D	Bone health, immune function	Sunlight, fortified milk, fatty fish
Calcium	Bone and tooth development	Dairy products, leafy greens, fortified cereals
Iron	Red blood cell production, energy	Meat, poultry, fish, fortified cereals, leafy greens
Zinc	Immune function, growth and development	Meat, poultry, seafood, beans, nuts, seeds
Omega-3 fatty acids	Brain and eye development	Fatty fish, flaxseeds, walnuts, chia seeds

CHAPTER 11
Physical Activity and Play

Scan QR code for more information on this chapter

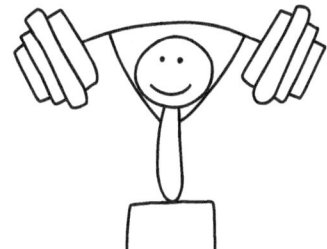

Physical Activity

Physical activity is any bodily movement produced by skeletal muscles that requires energy expenditure. It encompasses all types of movement, including leisure activities, transportation, work, and household chores. Physical activity is categorized by intensity: gentle, moderate, or vigorous. Moderate- and vigorous-intensity activities offer significant health benefits. Moderate-intensity activities increase heart rate by 50-60% above resting levels.

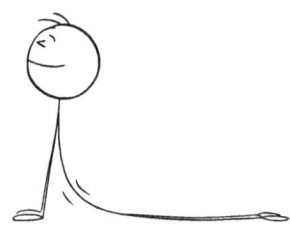

Physical activity is vital for children's **health, development,** and **well-being**. It strengthens bones, muscles, and lungs, improves coordination, balance, and flexibility, boosts the immune system, and helps maintain a healthy weight. Engaging in physical activity reduces the risk of type 2 diabetes, high blood pressure, anxiety, and depression. It also enhances sleep, concentration, and self-esteem.

90% of children do not meet CDC physical activity standards, affecting 50 million kids. Lack of physical activity hinders gross motor milestones, impacting fine motor skills, social-emotional development, and speech and language skills.

Engaging in physical activity plays a vital role in both play and learning. Peer interaction during play can enhance social-emotional growth by fostering skills like sharing, turn-taking, and cooperation. This interaction not only helps children form relationships within their families and communities but also enhances communication and language abilities through physical activity.

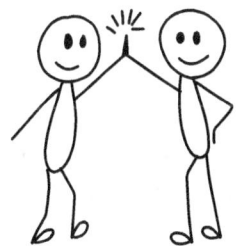

How active should children be?

Encouraging Babies to Stay Active

- It's important for babies to stay active daily in different ways, such as crawling.
- For non-crawling babies, promote physical activity through reaching, grasping, pulling, pushing, and moving their head, body, and limbs during daily activities and supervised floor play.
- Aim for 30 minutes of tummy time during awake periods throughout the day.

Once babies start moving, support them to be active in a safe and supervised play setting.

Physical Activity for Toddlers

- Toddlers need at least 180 minutes of physical activity daily.
- Activities should be spread throughout the day and include both light and energetic movements.
- Outdoor play is encouraged.

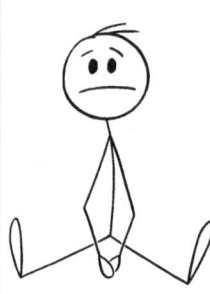

Children under 5 should not be inactive for long periods, except when they're asleep. Watching TV, travelling by car, bus or train, or being strapped into a stroller/car seat for long periods are not good for a child's health and development.

When children lack physical activity, they often spend time on screens. **Excessive screen time** can lead to obesity, sleep disorders, depression, anxiety, hinder emotional development, increase aggression, and impact overall mental health.

Physical Activity for Preschoolers

- Preschoolers are recommended to engage in a minimum of 180 minutes (3 hours) of diverse physical activities daily.
- Active and outdoor play distributed throughout the day. More activity is encouraged for better health.
- Within the 180 minutes, it is advised to have at least 60 minutes (1 hour) of moderate-to-vigorous intensity physical activity.

Increased **TV exposure** between 6-18 months linked to **emotional reactivity, aggression, and externalizing behaviors.** Higher screen time at 4 years associated with **lower emotional understanding** at 6 years. Having a TV in a child's bedroom at 6 years predicts lower emotional understanding at 8 years.

> **Computer use and video gaming**, but not television viewing, were shown to be connected with more **severe depressive symptoms** when looking at the effects of various types of screens. Video gaming, in particular, is correlated with the severity of anxiety
>
> Excessive screen usage **can also lead to problems in social-emotional development, including obesity, sleep disturbances, depression, and anxiety**. It can impair emotional comprehension, promote aggressive behavior, and hinder social and emotional competence.
>
> Muppalla SK, Vuppalapati S, Reddy Pulliahgaru A, Sreenivasulu H. *Effects of Excessive Screen Time on Child Development: An Updated Review and Strategies for Management.* Cureus. 2023 Jun 18;15

Computers & video games

The Negative Impact of Screens on Children's Development:

- Screens can impede attention span and focus development, affecting brain growth and processing of stimuli.

- Excessive screen time can hinder the learning of coping mechanisms and impulse control in children, resulting in reduced imagination and motivation.

- Exposure to screens can limit face-to-face interactions essential for understanding non-verbal cues and developing social skills, thereby affecting the development of empathy.

- Monitoring screen quality and interacting with children during screen time can help reduce negative effects; however, limiting or avoiding screen time in early childhood can be advantageous for long-term development.

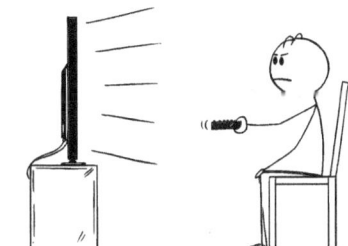

Screens Impacting Attention Span and Development in Children

- Children's success relies on their ability to concentrate and focus, which begins developing in their early years.

- To foster brain growth, children need essential stimuli from their environment and time to process it.

- The constant exposure to on-screen content affects children's attention span and focus negatively.

Limiting Impulses and Promoting Self-Reliance

- Boredom is essential for young children as it helps them cope with frustration and control impulses.
- Overstimulation by screens can hinder self-reliance, leading to frustration, and impeding imagination and motivation.

Reduced Empathy Due to Screen Time

- Screen time inhibits children's ability to learn social skills and read non-verbal cues necessary for empathy.
- Face-to-face interactions help young children understand emotions and develop empathy.
- Limiting screen time and focusing on quality content can help preserve children's emotional development and cognitive abilities.

Play

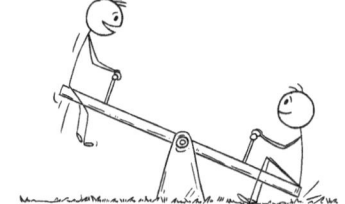

Play is a fundamental aspect of childhood development, recognized by organizations like NAEYC and the United Nations High Commission on Human Rights. It's not a frivolous activity but a crucial component of a child's growth. Play fosters self-discovery, relationships, and emotional well-being while promoting creativity, empathy, and resilience.

A lack of play can significantly hinder a child's development. It's essential to prioritize play in childhood to nurture well-rounded, content adults.

Play is a cornerstone of childhood development, supporting cognitive, physical, social, and emotional well-being. Through play, children unleash their creativity, enhance their imagination, and develop physical, cognitive, and emotional skills.

Healthy brain development is closely tied to play. It allows children to explore and engage with the world around them, overcoming fears, practicing adult roles, and collaborating with others. By mastering their surroundings, children build confidence and resilience, preparing them for future challenges.

Stages of Play

Play is a fundamental aspect of childhood development, evolving as children grow and mature.

Here are the primary stages of play:
1. Solitary Play (0-2 years)
- Description: Children play alone, often focusing on their own toys or activities.
- Benefits: Develops independence and self-awareness.

2. Parallel Play (2-3 years)
- Description: Children play side-by-side with others, often using the same toys but not interacting directly.
- Benefits: Encourages social awareness and observation of peers.

3. Associative Play (3-4 years)
- Description: Children play together, often sharing toys and engaging in similar activities but without a shared goal.
- Benefits: Fosters social skills and cooperation.

4. Cooperative Play (4+ years)
- Description: Children play together with a shared goal, taking on different roles and working together towards a common purpose.
- Benefits: Develops teamwork, problem-solving, and communication skills.

Note: These stages are general guidelines, and individual children may progress through them at different rates. It's important to support children at their developmental level and encourage them to explore different types of play.

Types of Play

Unoccupied Play
- **Description:** Children appear to be engaged in random movements or activities without a clear purpose.
- **Common in:** Early infancy

Independent Play / Solitary Play
- **Description:** Children play alone, often focusing on their own toys or activities.
- **Common in:** Early childhood, but can continue throughout development.

Symbolic Play
- **Description:** Children use objects or actions to represent something else, such as using a banana as a telephone.
- **Common in:** Preschool and early elementary years

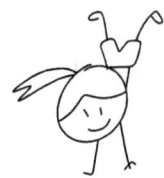 # Types of Play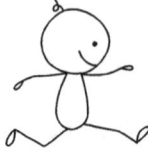

Onlooker Play
- **Description:** Children watch others play but do not participate.
- **Common in:** Toddlers and preschoolers

Parallel Play
- **Description:** Children play side-by-side, often using the same toys but not interacting directly.
- **Common in**: Early childhood

Associative Play
- **Description:** Children play together, often sharing toys and engaging in similar activities but without a shared goal.
- **Common in:** Preschool and early elementary years

Cooperative Play
- **Description:** Children play together with a shared goal, taking on different roles and working together towards a common purpose.
- **Common in:** Elementary school and beyond

Dramatic or Fantasy Play
- **Description:** Children pretend to be someone or something else, often using props or imaginary scenarios.
- **Common in:** Preschool and early elementary years

Physical Play
- **Description:** Involves physical activity, such as running, jumping, climbing, and dancing.
- **Common in:** All ages, but particularly important for young children's development.

Remember: These are general guidelines, and children may engage in different types of play at various stages of development. It's essential to support a variety of play experiences to promote healthy growth and development.

> In previous generations, play used to be a child-led, unstructured activity. Nowadays, many children experience play as supervised and tightly organized, which greatly influences their physical, cognitive, social, and emotional development.

think about......

- Children should master foundational skills to reach their highest level of function.

- Without a strong foundation, learning can be difficult!

- There's more to sensory challenges than just being bothered by noise. Understanding the different senses and how they can impact the child is key.

- If children lack core strength, they tire easily and struggle to pay attention while sitting up straight.

How do I help a child improve core strength..

Here are some fun and engaging activities to help your child improve their core strength:
Play-Based Activities:
- **Animal poses:** Encourage your child to imitate animals like a cat, frog, or bird. These poses engage various core muscles.
- **Balancing games:** Have your child balance on one leg, a narrow beam, or a wobble board.
- **Tummy time:** Encourage tummy time activities, such as crawling, reaching for toys, or propping up on their forearms.
- **Obstacle courses:** Set up obstacle courses with tunnels, climbing structures, and balance beams to challenge their core muscles.

Specific Exercises:
- **Plank:** Have your child hold a plank position, keeping their body straight from head to heels.
- **Superman:** Lie on their stomach and simultaneously lift their arms, legs, and chest off the ground.
- **Bicycle crunches:** Lie on their back, bring knees toward chest, and alternate touching opposite elbow to knee.
- **Boat pose:** Sit with knees bent, lean back slightly, and lift feet off the ground.
- **Bird-dog:** Get on all fours and extend opposite arm and leg simultaneously.

Remember to make these activities fun and engaging for your child. Start with shorter durations and gradually increase the time as they become stronger.

Additionally, consider incorporating core-strengthening exercises into everyday activities:
- **Carrying heavy objects:** Let them help carry groceries or laundry baskets.
- **Playing outside:** Activities like climbing trees, swimming, or riding a bike can naturally strengthen core muscles.

By incorporating these activities into your child's routine, you can help them develop strong core muscles, which will benefit their overall balance, coordination, and posture.

Gross Motor Milestones in Children

Gross motor skills involve the large muscles of the body, such as those in the legs, arms, and torso. Developing these skills is essential for everyday activities like walking, running, jumping, and throwing.

Key Gross Motor Milestones:

Infancy (0-12 months):
- Lifts head while lying on stomach
- Rolls over
- Sits with support
- Crawls
- Stands with support
- Walks with assistance

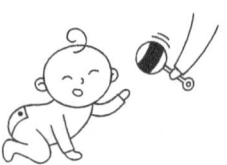

Toddlerhood (1-3 years):
- Walks independently
- Runs
- Kicks a ball
- Climbs stairs
- Jumps
- Pedals a tricycle

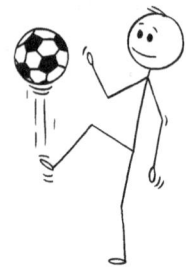

Preschool (3-5 years):
- Runs smoothly
- Hops on one foot
- Skips
- Throws and catches a ball
- Rides a bike with training wheels

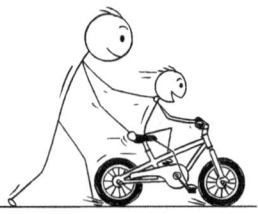

Elementary School (6-12 years):
- Continues to refine running, jumping, and throwing skills
- Develops balance and coordination
- Participates in sports and other physical activities

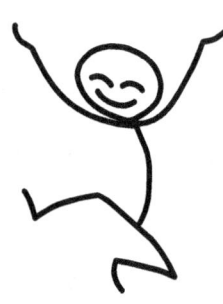

Remember, these are general milestones, and individual children may develop at different rates. If you have concerns about your child's gross motor development, consult with a healthcare professional.

To support your child's gross motor development, encourage physical activity and provide opportunities for practice. This can include activities like playing outside, swimming, dancing, and participating in sports.

CHAPTER 12
Treatment, Strategies and Activities

Scan QR code for more information on this chapter

When a child exhibits developmental delays, **occupational therapy (OT), physical therapy (PT),** and **speech therapy** can play crucial roles in addressing their specific needs.

- **OT** focuses on improving daily living skills, fine motor skills, and sensory processing.

- **PT** helps develop gross motor skills, balance, and coordination.

- **Speech therapy** addresses communication, language, and swallowing difficulties.

By working together, these therapies can provide comprehensive support to help children overcome challenges, reach their full potential, and participate more fully in their daily lives. It is important to learn what services children in your care receive in order to incorporate it into your daily activities in your environment.

Strategies, treatments, and activities are often used interchangeably, but it's crucial to recognize the distinctions among these terms.

- **"Treatment"** is typically associated with medical professionals who provide therapy prescribed by a physician.
- Therapists offer **strategies** to families, caregivers, and teachers to address specific concerns throughout the day.
- **Activities,** on the other hand, are utilized by therapists, teachers, or families to teach new skills or engage in tasks.

Direct therapy interventions are carried out under a physician's guidance. A licensed therapist evaluates the need for therapy, plans treatment, and administers direct services. These services vary based on factors like the type of therapy and the child's needs and parental input.

- Therapists create **strategies** tailored to individual children to aid in their overall development.
- Caregivers implement **activities** to support children's development, either individually or in groups.

Direct interventions are personalized after a thorough evaluation of each child. Such interventions are not discussed generally, as therapists devise a specific care plan. Specific strategies and activities will be outlined in subsequent chapters.

Schedules

Children thrive on predictability and routine. Consistent daily schedules and step-by-step routines provide a sense of control and security. In both group care settings and homes, these structures help children:

- **Feel in control:** Predictability reduces anxiety and fosters a sense of agency.

- **Understand expectations:** Clear routines minimize confusion and challenging behaviors.

- **Communicate effectively:** Visual schedules provide a concrete representation of tasks, aiding understanding.

A visual schedule is a series of pictures representing a sequence of activities or events. It breaks down tasks into simple steps, providing visual cues for each routine stage. By combining pictures, photographs, graphics, and words, visual schedules guide children in understanding where they should be, what they should do, and when they should do it.

> Schedule use must be taught. Do not assume just because you have made the schedule that the child or children know what it is. Explain to the child or children why they have a schedule. Make sure they understand the schedule. Make sure they know what each picture refers too. The schedule needs to be in the same place all the time or available at all times.

Just like adults, children thrive on predictability and familiarity in their daily routines, which help them feel confident and secure. Consistent schedules and step-by-step routines provide children with a sense of control and structure throughout their day. Here are some benefits of implementing schedules and routines for children both in group care settings and at home:

- Feeling in control of their environment
- Understanding what is expected of them leads to better compliance with adult requests
- Clear instructions on what to do rather than what not to do can reduce challenging behaviors
- Visual aids, such as photographs or charts, help children comprehend expectations and minimize challenging behaviors
- Visual schedules, using pictures to depict activity steps, can be used to teach routines like preparing for school at home
- Visual schedules break down tasks into manageable steps and offer visual cues for each stage of a routine
- By combining pictures, photos, graphics, and words, visual schedules effectively guide children on where to be, what to do, and when to do it

Establishing a Solid Foundation for All Age Groups

Routines play a crucial role in every stage of childhood, from infancy to pre-adolescence. Here's how routines aid children at different stages:

- **Newborns and Infants (0-1 Year):** Establish a sense of security and predictability for newborns and infants through consistent sleep, feeding, and play routines. This helps regulate their sleep patterns and promotes overall development.

- **Toddlers (1-3 Years):** Toddlers benefit from routines that offer structure and predictability, helping them anticipate events. Consistent schedules for meals, naps, and activities support their growing independence and foster a sense of control.

- **Preschoolers (3-5 Years):** Routines provide predictability and structure for preschoolers. Daily schedules for learning, playtime, and rest help them navigate their day confidently and enhance social skills through group interactions.

- **Early School Age (6-8 Years):** Routines aid academic and social growth in early elementary school children. Consistent homework times, extracurricular activities, and bedtime routines help them manage responsibilities and balance activities.

- **Older School Age (9-12 Years):** Older elementary school children benefit from routines that promote responsibility and self-management. Structured schedules for homework, chores, and leisure activities help them develop time-management skills and prepare for more complex duties.

How to make and use picture/ written schedules.

Visual Schedule Materials:
- Paint sticks: A vertical surface for displaying pictures or symbols.
- Bulletin boards: Ideal for classroom schedules.
- Folders: Provide privacy for individual schedules.
- Binders: Offer both privacy and functionality for older children.
- Clip art or photographs: Visual representations of items and tasks.
- Written directions: For older children who can read, use clear, concise sentences and bullet points.

Choose a font that is easy for the child to read and tailor the schedule to their age and developmental level.

If the child needs a pictures schedule there are many choices. Programs that provide both pictures and templets are available for a fee. One examples of such programs is Boardmaker by Mayor Johnson http://www.mayer-johnson.com/boardmaker-software-family.

How to Create a Visual Schedule

Creating a visual schedule tailored to your specific needs is essential for organizing your classroom, curriculum, and supporting children's development.

Here's a detailed guide on making a visual schedule:

- **Step 1:** Choose a routine to focus on, such as a mid-morning snack time or end-of-day activity.

- **Step 2:** Divide the activity into manageable steps.

- **Step 3:** Determine the duration of the schedule, starting with simpler tasks and progressing to more complex ones based on the children's abilities.

- **Step 4:** Select appropriate visual aids like photographs, graphics, symbols, and text with images. Personalize the visuals to make them more engaging, including pictures of each child completing the steps.

- **Step 5:** Create your visual schedule using programs like Microsoft Word, Publisher, PowerPoint, or graphic design software like Adobe Photoshop and Canva.

- **Step 6:** Introduce the visual schedule to the children, explaining its purpose and how to use it effectively.

- **Step 7:** Encourage and acknowledge children's efforts when following the schedule or completing tasks independently by praising their accomplishments.

Plan for the unexpected

Preparing for the Unexpected: Incorporating a Change Symbol

Visual schedules can be disrupted by unexpected changes, leading to meltdowns. To address this, introduce a change symbol to represent schedule modifications.

Choosing a Symbol:

- **Options:** Consider using a yield sign, yellow light, or a specific color or shape.
- **Introduction:** Teach the child what the symbol represents through a social story or a fun, unexpected change in the schedule.
- **Consistency:** Use the same symbol each time there's a schedule change.

Implementing the Change Symbol:

- **Early notification:** Place the symbol on the schedule when a change becomes known.
- **Point out the change:** Alert the child to the schedule modification using the symbol.

By using a change symbol, you can help children anticipate and adapt to unexpected changes in their routine, reducing anxiety and promoting flexibility.

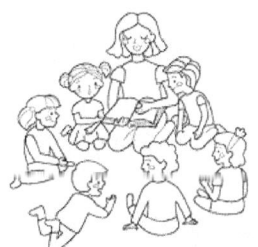
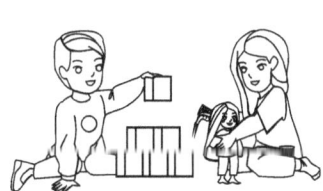
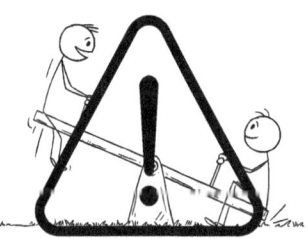

Circle time   Center time   Outside

Timers

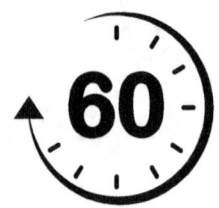

Introduce the Timer in a Fun Way
- Start by introducing the timer with a more enjoyable approach, rather than as a task.
- Use it when the activity following the timer ending is something fun for your child.
- Place the timer where your child can easily see it to turn the countdown into a fun activity.

Explain the Timer Function
- Get on your child's level, make eye contact, and explain that when the timer goes off, it's time to switch activities.
- Use an affirmative tone and eye contact to communicate the transition.
- For non-verbal children, a kind tone and eye contact are sufficient.
- For verbal children, confirm their understanding of the upcoming change.

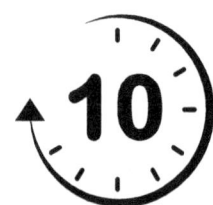

Maintain a Positive Tone
- Upon the timer signal, use a positive, reassuring tone to announce the switch in activities.
- Acknowledge your child's emotions while setting the boundary.
- Example: "I understand you enjoy playing with blocks, but now it's puzzle time."

Start with One or Two Transition Periods
- Begin gradually by introducing the timer during one transition per day.
- Once your child grasps the concept, expand its use to challenging transitions like bedtime.
- Consistency is key to effectively integrating timers into daily routines.

3 Strategies to Incorporate Timers into Daily Life
- Visual timers require time and consistency for successful implementation.
- Use a positive tone to communicate boundaries and expectations related to the timer.
- Acknowledge and praise positive behavior instead of focusing solely on negative aspects through discipline.

Remember: Using a timer requires patience and consistency. Focus on positive reinforcement and avoid using it as a punishment tool.

Tip #1: Use Timers for Transitions

- **Introduce the timer:** Explain that the timer will signal the end of an activity.
- **Set expectations:** Clearly communicate the duration of the activity.
- **Positive reinforcement:** Praise your child for following the timer.

Example: "Let's watch TV for 20 minutes. When the timer goes off, it's time to turn off the TV."

Tip #2: Foster Independent Play

- **Use the timer as a tool:** Explain that you need to finish a task and suggest independent play.
- **Set expectations:** Clearly communicate the duration of the independent play time.
- **Positive reinforcement:** Praise your child for playing independently.

Example: "I need to finish dinner. Can you play independently until the timer goes off? Then we can play together."

Tip #3: Increase Activity Duration

- **Start small:** Begin with shorter durations and gradually increase the time.
- **Positive reinforcement:** Praise your child for completing the activity.
- **Gradual progression:** Increase the time incrementally over several days.

Example: "Let's try sitting quietly for 15 minutes. If you can do it, we'll try 20 minutes tomorrow."

Remember: Consistency, positive reinforcement, and patience are key to successfully using timers with children.

Sand timers: Provide a visual cue that can be helpful for some children.

Digital timers: On tablets or phones, these can be easily controlled and turned off if the child becomes fixated on watching.

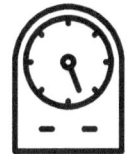

Desktop timers: Offer various time options but may have distracting sounds.

Choose a timer that is appropriate for your child's age, preferences, and needs. **Consider their visual and auditory sensitivities when making a selection.**

Morning Schedules: Examples

For young children, use simple pictures only. You can place pictures on a card or use magnets and a magnet board. For older children you should include the words and may include times.

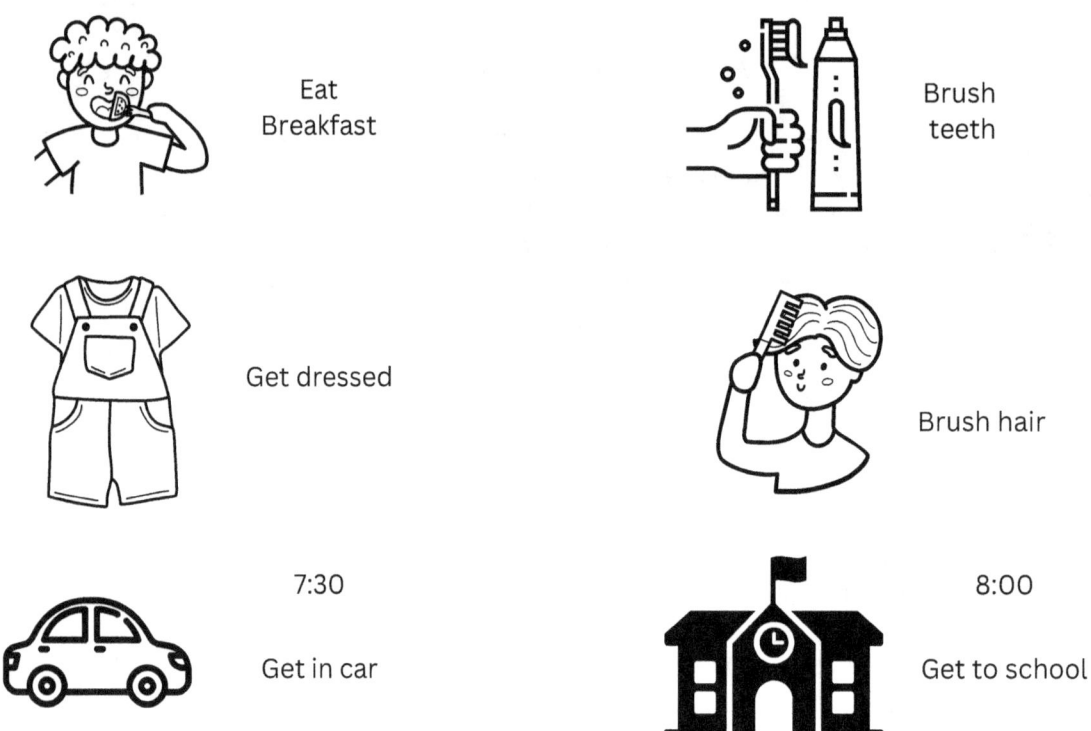

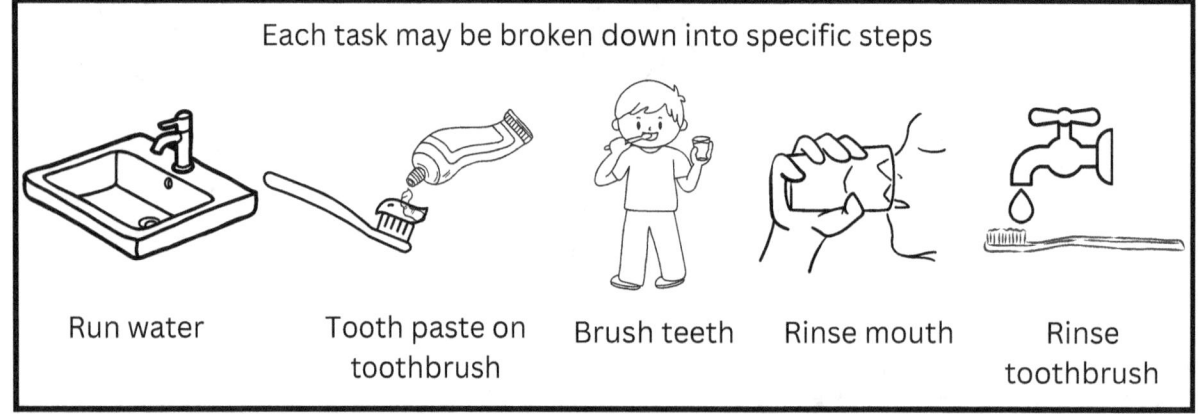

Video Modeling

Video Modeling: A Powerful Teaching Tool

Video modeling is an evidence-based practice that involves students watching a model perform a target skill on video and then practicing the skill themselves. This technique can be used to teach a wide range of skills, including communication, daily living, social, and academic skills.

Research has shown that video modeling is effective for learners from early childhood through middle school. While there is limited research on high school students, it may also be beneficial at this age level.

Implementing Video Modeling:

1. **Identify the target skill:** Determine the specific behavior or skill you want to improve.
2. **Gather baseline data:** Collect data on the current frequency and severity of the target behavior. For example, if the issue is interrupting conversations, record the number of interruptions per day over a two-week period.
3. **Create the video model:** Record a video of someone (a peer, teacher, or adult) demonstrating the desired behavior. The model should be clear, concise, and engaging.
4. **Show the video:** Have the student watch the video multiple times.
5. **Provide practice opportunities:** Allow the student to practice the skill with guidance and support.
6. **Monitor progress:** Continue to collect data and make adjustments to the video model or support as needed.

By following these steps, you can effectively use video modeling to improve student behavior and skills.

Choosing a Video Modeling Approach

There are four types of video modeling:

- **Basic video modeling:** A familiar or unfamiliar person demonstrates the target skill.
- **Video self-modeling:** The child is the model, showcasing positive behaviors or handling difficult situations.
- **Point-of-view modeling:** The video is filmed from the student's perspective.
- **Video prompting:** Demonstrates each step of a task sequentially.

Creating a Video Model:

1. **Obtain parent permission** if using student models.
2. **Write a script:** Develop a clear and concise script for the video.
3. **Record the video:** Keep it simple and concise, ideally between two and four minutes.

Using a Video Model:

- **Timing:** Show the video daily or at specific times related to the target behavior.
- **Data collection:** Track changes in the target behavior.
- **Fading:** Gradually reduce video viewing frequency as the behavior improves.

Remember to tailor the video modeling approach to the student's individual needs and preferences.

Stories

Social Stories: A Powerful Tool for Autism

Social Stories are a trademarked strategy developed by child pediatrician Dr. Carol Gray in the early 1990s. Initially created for autistic children, these narratives illustrate social situations and problems, helping individuals with autism understand social norms and communicate effectively.

To be considered a true Social Story, it must meet ten specific criteria:

Here's a brief summary of the ten criteria:

1. **Positive tone:** The story should be written in a positive and supportive manner.
2. **Learner's perspective:** The story should be told from the child's point of view.
3. **Descriptive language:** Use clear and concise language to describe the situation.
4. **Explanation of ambiguous terms:** Define any unfamiliar words or concepts.
5. **Focus on "can do" statements**: Emphasize what the child can do rather than what they can't.
6. **Sequential order:** Present information in a logical and understandable sequence.
7. **Visual supports:** Incorporate visuals (e.g., pictures, symbols) to enhance understanding.
8. **Individualized:** Tailor the story to the child's specific needs and abilities.
9. **Repetition:** Use repetition to reinforce key concepts.
10. **Collaboration:** Involve the child and their family in the development and implementation of the Social Story.

By following these guidelines, Social Stories can be a valuable tool for supporting individuals with autism in navigating social interactions.

Personal Stories: Tailored Support for Children

Personal stories are narratives that provide children with specific information about situations, concerns, or events. Unlike Social Stories, they do not require strict adherence to ten specific criteria.

Creating Personal Stories:

- **Format:** Choose a book or digital format.
- **Language:** Use age-appropriate language that the child can easily understand.
- **Length:** Keep the story concise to maintain the child's attention.
- **Visuals:** Include relevant pictures, possibly featuring the child themselves.

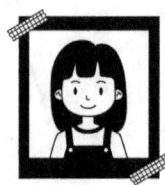

Example: Preparing for a Field Trip

A personal story about a field trip can help children anticipate and manage the excitement, sensory overload, and new experiences involved. Reading the story daily before the trip can ease anxiety and set expectations.

Tips for Creating Personal Stories:

- Use simple language and clear visuals.
- Relate the story to the child's personal experiences.
- Focus on the child's feelings and emotions.
- Provide positive messages and encouragement.

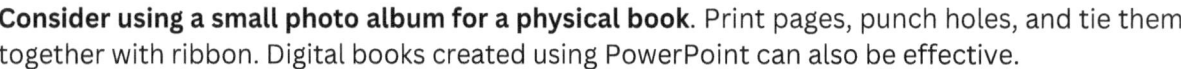

Consider using a small photo album for a physical book. Print pages, punch holes, and tie them together with ribbon. Digital books created using PowerPoint can also be effective.

By creating personalized stories, you can provide children with valuable support and help them navigate challenging situations.

Going to the dentist

Sometimes I need to go to the Dentist.

The Dentist is the person that makes sure our teeth are healthy.

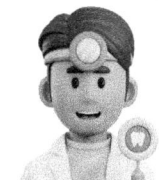

When I go to the Dentist, I will sit in the waiting room and wait my turn.

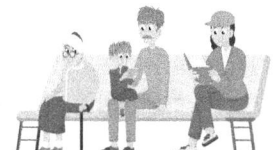

When my name is called, I will walk back and sit in the Dentist chair.

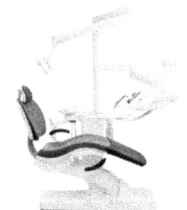

The dential assistant will put a bib on me and turn on more lights to help the dentist see in my mouth.
I can close my eyes, if the lights are too bright.

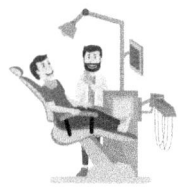

When the dentist ask me to open my mouth, I will open wide and lay very still while he looks at my teeth.

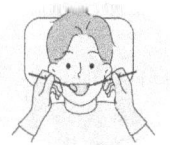

The dentist may use different tools that sound funny. If I get scared I can ask for a break.

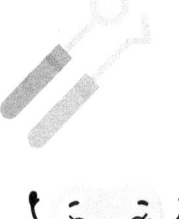

After my teeth brushed, I will be all done. My teeth will be all clean.

Using books

Using Books to Teach Social Emotional Skills

Books can be powerful tools for teaching children about social situations, emotions, and appropriate behaviors.

Here are some tips on how to use books effectively:

1. **Choose age-appropriate books:** Select books that are tailored to your child's age and reading level.
2. **Discuss the characters and their emotions:** Talk about the characters' feelings, actions, and the consequences of their choices.
3. **Relate the story to your child's experiences:** Connect the story to real-life situations your child might encounter.
4. **Encourage open-ended questions:** Ask questions that promote critical thinking and discussion.
5. **Role-play the story: Act** out the characters and scenarios from the book.
6. **Explore different perspectives:** Discuss the story from multiple characters' viewpoints.
7. **Practice social skills:** Use the book as a springboard for practicing social skills, such as sharing, taking turns, and being kind.

Here are some examples of books that can be used to teach social skills:

- "The Very Hungry Caterpillar" by Eric Carle: Teaches about patience, waiting, and making choices.

- "The Mitten" by Jan Brett: Teaches about sharing, friendship, and unexpected outcomes.

- "How to Be a Friend" by Jane O'Connor: Teaches about making friends, being kind, and resolving conflicts.

- "The Berenstain Bears" series: Covers a variety of social situations, such as sharing, taking turns, and being helpful.

By incorporating books into your child's learning experience, you can help them develop essential social skills and better understand the world around them.

Weighted Vest and Weighted Lap Blanket

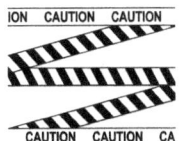 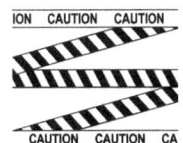

Who Should Avoid Using Weighted Blankets?

- Infants, toddlers, or very young children should avoid using weighted blankets due to the risk of pellets or glass beads falling out, posing a choking hazard, and the possibility of the heavy blanket covering their face during sleep.

- If you have sleep apnea, breathing difficulties, or any chronic health condition, it is advisable to consult your doctor before using a weighted blanket.

- Weighted blankets should never be used with children unable to physically remove the blanket.

Prior to allowing your child to sleep under a weighted blanket, seek advice from their pediatrician or therapist, especially if the child has epilepsy, breathing or heart issues, skin allergies, blood circulation problems, or struggles to remove the blanket independently.

Weighted lap blankets are another option to provide proprioceptive input to children. This is simply a small weighted pad that is placed in the child's lap. Use ONLY under the supervision of an Occupational Therapist who can assist in the proper weight. Too much weight can result in over stimulation and/or injury.

Deep pressure, provided through weighted vests or blankets, can be highly beneficial for children with autism, sensory integration disorder, ADHD, and other neurological disorders. By stimulating the muscles and joints, these tools can help children integrate sensory information, reduce anxiety, improve focus, and enhance learning abilities. Based on the sensory integration framework, the added weight or pressure provides the child with unconscious information from their muscles and joints.

There are no definitive guidelines for the ideal weight of a weighted vest. A common starting point is 5% of the child's body weight. However, it's essential to observe the child's response and make adjustments accordingly.

Consult with an occupational or physical therapist before using a weighted vest.
Weighted vests should NOT be worn for prolonged periods of time. Some therapist report it is ok to wear a minimum of 20 minutes and a maximum of two hours.

> **Please understand that it is IMPORTANT that you should never use a weighted blanket just because. ALWAYS speak with an experienced health care professional first. You can cause more harm than good.**

Quiet or Safe spaces

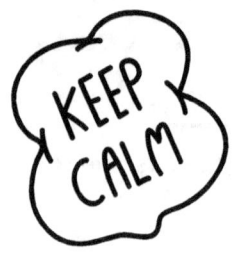

A quiet or safe space is not a time-out space.
- It's intended for calming down, reducing anxiety, or seeking safety.
- This space should be **separate and used independently** when needed.
- It's not about isolation but providing a safe haven from overwhelming environments.
- The child may choose to be alone or with a caregiver.

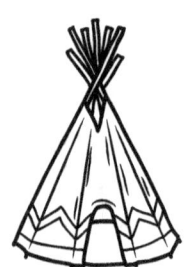

The space should be simple, safe, and easily accessible.
- Consider a pop-up tent, cardboard box, or sheet over a table.
- Include a favorite toy and calming items.
- Avoid clutter.
- Soft lighting and calming music can be beneficial, but ensure they are out of reach to prevent accidents.
- A book about emotions can also be helpful.

Teach your child about the quiet space when they are calm.
- Explain its purpose and share a personal story.
- You and your child can even name the space together.

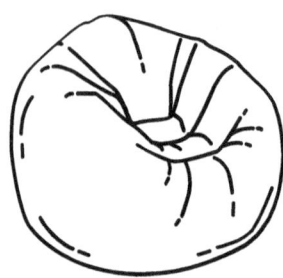

When you notice your child becoming upset, ask if they'd like to use the quiet space.
- If they refuse, respect their decision.
- Our goal is to teach, not force.
- If the child continues to escalate, identify their emotions and behaviors.
- Explain the connection between their actions and the need for a break.
- Offer to accompany them and engage in a calming activity.

If the child becomes upset quickly or resists going to the quiet space, you may need to gently guide them.

After calming down, provide positive feedback to encourage future use of the quiet space.

Movement Activities

Structured Movement Activities
To avoid overstimulation, incorporate a variety of structured movement activities that balance high-energy and calm moments. Combine fast-paced movements with slower, calming exercises.

Duration: Adjust the activity duration based on the child's age and tolerance. Younger children may benefit from shorter sessions (5-10 minutes), while older children can handle longer durations (15-20 minutes).

Music Integration: Use music to enhance the experience and provide a rhythmic structure for movements. Choose upbeat music for energetic activities and calming tunes for relaxation.

Remember: The goal is to create a balanced and enjoyable experience that promotes physical health, emotional regulation, and social interaction.

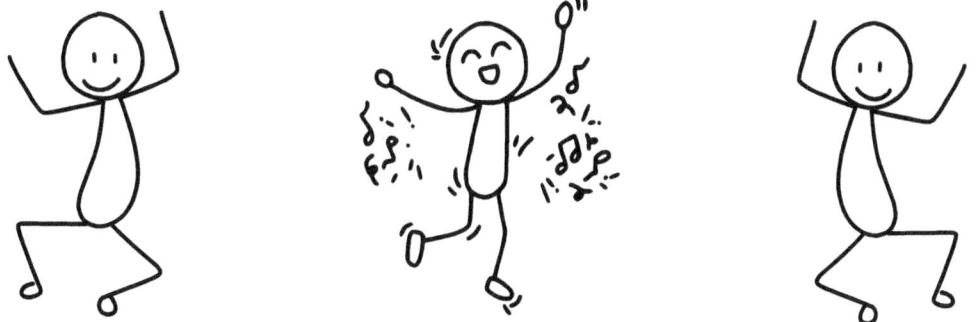

To keep children interested, incorporate a variety of movement activities:

- **Songs with actions:** For younger children, use classic songs like "Head, Shoulders, Knees, and Toes" or "The Hokey Pokey."
- **Games:** Older children may enjoy musical chairs or dance-offs.
- **Props:** Add scarves, ribbons, or instruments for tactile exploration.

Create a Safe Environment:
- **Space:** Ensure ample space for movement without the risk of injury.
- **Observation:** Monitor children for signs of fatigue or overstimulation.
- **Calming activities:** Prepare gentle stretching or deep breathing exercises for wind-down.

By offering a diverse range of movement activities, you can create a balanced and enjoyable experience that promotes physical health, emotional regulation, and social interaction.

Here is a list of our favorite activities

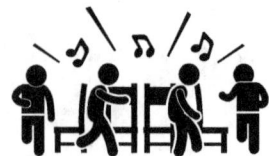

Musical Chairs – This classic game is a great way to get kids moving and groove to some tunes!

Hokey Pokey – Another classic that is sure to get kids moving, shaking, and giggling!

Balloon Bash – This game is sure to be a hit with the kiddos! They will love trying to keep the
balloons from hitting the ground.

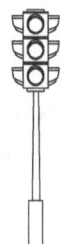

Red Light, Green Light – This is a great game for helping kids with following directions and motor skills.

Simon Says – A classic game that kids always love! This is a great way to get them to listen and follow directions.

Mother May I? – Another classic game that is perfect for getting kids moving. They will love trying to reach the finish line first.

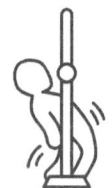

The limbo – How low can you go? This game is great for kids to practice their balance and flexibility.

Dance Party – Crank up the music and let the kids loose! This is a great way to get them moving and burning off some energy.

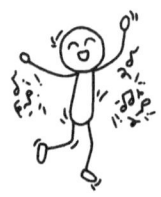

Freeze Dance – This game is always a hit with kids! They will love dancing around and then freezing when the music stops.

Duck, Duck, Goose – This is a great game for kids to run around and have some silly fun!

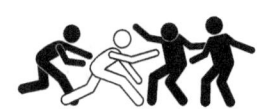

Tag- A simple game that can be played anywhere, Tag is a great way to get kids running around.

Hide and Seek – A classic game that is sure to get kids moving, Hide and Seek is a great way to get kids up and active.

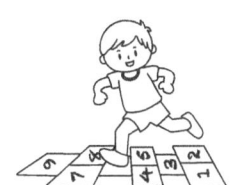
Hopscotch – A classic game that never goes out of style, Hopscotch is a great way to get kids moving.

Obstacle Course – A great way to get kids moving and thinking, an Obstacle Course is a great way to get kids up and moving around.

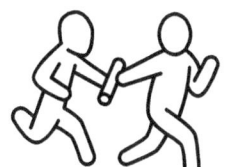
Red Rover – This is a great game for kids to play in a group. They will love trying to run and break through the line.

Relay Races – This is a great way to get kids moving and working together as a team.

Treasure/Scavenger Hunt – This is a great game for kids to use their problem-solving skills while they move around looking for the treasure.

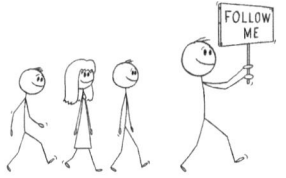
Follow the Leader – This game is great for groups of kids! They will have to follow the leader and do what they do.

Hot Potato – Another great game for groups of kids! They will have to work together to pass the potato around without dropping it.

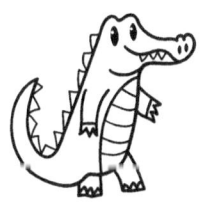
Please Mr. Crocodile, Can I Cross? – Another classic but oh-so-fun game! They will have to work together to get across the crocodile without getting eaten.

Movement strategies in the classroom

- Allow the child to stand. A door mat or tape can be placed on the floor to ensure boundaries.

- Have the child take a note to another teacher or to the office. This allows the child a few minutes to move with a purpose.

- Allow the child to lay down (on stomach)

Movement for the entire class must be structured.

- March in place or march around the room.

- Stand up, sit down. Have the entire class stand up then sit down 5 times.

- Head, Shoulder, Knees and Toes

Noise Reducing Headphones

Here's a breakdown of the differences between noise cancellation and noise reduction headphones:

- **Noise Cancellation Headphones:** These headphones use advanced technology to actively reduce external noise by producing sound waves that counteract the noise. This creates a quieter environment for the listener.

- **Noise Reduction Headphones:** These headphones rely on passive noise cancellation, which simply blocks out external noise by creating a physical barrier between the listener's ears and the environment.

In essence, noise cancellation headphones offer a more effective and immersive listening experience.

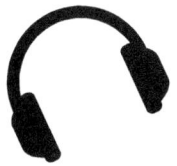 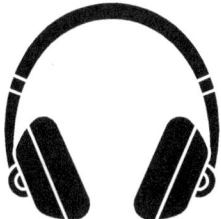 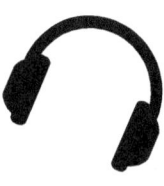

Noise-reducing headphones can be beneficial for children in several ways:

1. **Sensory Sensitivity:** For children with sensory sensitivities or sensory processing disorders, noise reduction headphones can help reduce overwhelming auditory stimuli, making it easier to focus and learn.
2. **Noise Pollution:** In noisy environments, such as schools or crowded areas, noise reduction headphones can help protect children's hearing from excessive noise exposure.
3. **Concentration:** By reducing background noise, noise reduction headphones can help children concentrate better on tasks that require focus, such as studying or completing homework.
4. **Sleep:** For children who have trouble sleeping due to noise, noise reduction headphones can create a quieter environment, promoting better sleep quality.
5. **Travel:** When traveling, noise reduction headphones can help children relax and enjoy their journey by reducing the noise of airplanes, trains, or cars.

It's important to note that noise reduction headphones should not be used as a substitute for professional evaluation or treatment for sensory processing disorders or hearing problems. If you have concerns about your child's hearing or sensory sensitivity, consult with a healthcare professional.

Space

Children can become overwhelmed, frustrated, and tired. When this happens, they may need a break to calm down or recharge. Allowing them to say "I need a minute" (or use their own words) is an excellent way to teach coping strategies.

Providing space and time for self-regulation does not mean isolating the child. It's an opportunity to calm down and then rejoin their daily activities. **Avoid using "time-out" as a punishment.**

During this quiet time, music can be soothing, but screen time should be avoided. The goal is to help the child relax and regain their composure.

Remember: By allowing children to express their need for a break and providing a supportive environment, we are teaching them valuable coping skills that will benefit them throughout their lives.

Music

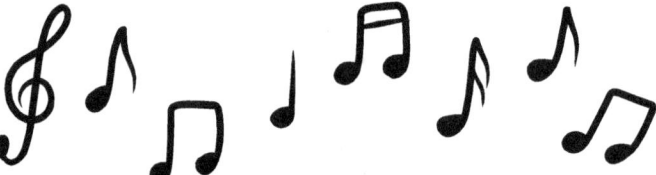

Exposure to music can positively influence a child's behavior, regardless of the musical style. Music strengthens the corpus callosum, the bridge between the brain's hemispheres. This improved connection enhances a child's ability to regulate mood, emotions, and behavior.

Music's Impact on Early Development

Music offers numerous benefits for babies and toddlers, including:

- **Language development:** Exposure to music helps babies develop speech skills by stimulating their auditory senses and encouraging vocalization.

- **Motor skills:** Music provides opportunities for physical movement, supporting motor development and coordination.\

- **Emotional well-being:** Music can soothe and calm babies and toddlers, promoting emotional regulation.

- **Parent-child bonding:** Shared musical experiences release oxytocin, a bonding hormone, strengthening the parent-child relationship.

By incorporating music into your child's early experiences, you can lay the foundation for a lifelong love of music and a host of cognitive benefits.

Music: A Versatile Tool for Childcare Settings

Music can be used in various ways to enhance the classroom environment and support children's development.

- **Mood and Atmosphere:** Fast-paced music can increase activity levels, while slow music can promote relaxation.
- **Language and Following Directions:** Music with lyrics encourages singing and following directions.
- **Focus and Immersion:** Headphones provide a more immersive listening experience, reducing distractions and enhancing focus.
- **Stress Reduction:** Classical music has been shown to reduce stress, anxiety, and heart rate.
- **Improved Listening Skills:** Consistent exposure to classical music can enhance listening abilities in children.
- **Cognitive Benefits:** The calming effects of classical music can lead to clearer thinking and boosted creativity.

By incorporating music into your childcare setting, you can create a more engaging, relaxing, and stimulating environment for children.

Sleep Strategies

Routine:
- This is a great time to use a visual schedule. Use pictures to identify each step of the bed time routine.
- Use music or a song to cue the start of the bedtime routine.
- Have the same bed time each night
- Have the same wake up time each morning

Room color:
Color can be calming or chaotic. Super bright colors are stimulating. Using high contrasting colors are stimulating as well. Choose solid colors or simple patterns for the child's room to enhance a relaxed atmosphere. Using lamps or a dimmer also helps encourage relaxation.

Room organization:
Too many toys is too much stimulation. Organization creates calm. Use baskets or boxes to put toys away and discourage temptation to get up and play.

Bedding:
Does your child have a preference for the texture of their sheets ? Sheets may seem itchy, hot or heavy.
- Try cooling sheets if your child is hot.
- Use fleece sheets for softness.
- Lycra sheets provide a snug fit and are cool
- Quilts are heavy and may provide a calming affect

Music:
Slow instrumental music is soothing. Use an audio player not a video / screen.

Lights:
Night lights provide a dim but secure light for children. Children who have become accustomed to screen time at bedtime may benefit for a small projector that illuminates the ceiling or a wall.

Bedtime Story:
Bedtime stories are a wonderful way to connect with your child and provide a sense of safety. You do not have to read the story word for word but some children may prefer that.

Alarm clock:
An alarm clock for kids can help teach healthy sleep schedules. A toddler alarm clock can provide a visual cue that it's still nighttime and everyone should sleep. Having an alarm to wake up can provide the child a sense of independence.

Weighted blanket

Weighted blankets should never be used for infants or children that are unable to independently remove the blanket.

The rule of thumb for use of weighted blankets is 10% of the child's body weight.

Nutritional Strategies

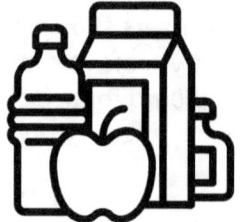

Meal times / Routines:

Feeding schedules help a child to develop regular patterns of appetite and ensure a child is well nourished throughout the day. In general, young children should have three meals and two to three snacks each day.

Children should sit with the family at meals. Research shows that sharing a fun family meal is good for the spirit, brain and health of all family members. Recent studies link regular family meals with the kinds of behaviors that parents want for their children: higher grade-point averages, resilience, and self-esteem. Additionally, family meals are linked to lower rates of substance abuse, teen pregnancy, eating disorders, and depression.

Make food fun
- Use a cookie cutter to cut out sandwiches
- Make animals or shapes with fruits and vegetables
- Use fun shapes of colored plates and utensil

Let children help
- Let children help choose a meal
- Let them help you shop for items at the grocery store
- Engage them in cooking. Let them help stir items or assist in a safe way

Make nutritional changes
- Decrease the number of sodas and juice and increase water intake
    - Add water to sodas and juice to make the transition easier
- Begin offering fruit as a snack
- Decrease highly processed foods

Slowly introduce different foods.

- Introduce a variety of foods from different cultures to expand their palate.
- Offer new foods alongside familiar favorites to make them more approachable.
- Be patient and persistent; it can take multiple exposures for a child to accept a new food.

Encourage mindful eating

- Teach children to listen to their hunger and fullness cues.
- Encourage them to eat slowly and savor each bite.
- Create a calm eating environment free from distractions like TV or electronic devices.

Model healthy eating habits

- Show enthusiasm for trying new foods and maintaining a balanced diet.
- Demonstrate portion control and the importance of eating a variety of food groups.
- Be a role model by making healthy choices yourself.

Celebrate successes

- Praise children for trying new foods, even if they don't like them right away.
- Celebrate small milestones to build positive associations with healthy eating.
- Keep a food adventure journal to track new foods they've tried and liked.

By incorporating these strategies, you can create a positive and nourishing mealtime experience that supports your child's overall development and well-being.

Chores

Age-Appropriate Chores for Children

Assigning age-appropriate chores can help children develop responsibility, independence, and a sense of belonging. Here are some chore ideas based on age:

Toddlers (1-3 years):
- Put toys away
- Place clothes in the hamper
- Help set the table
- Wipe up spills
- Dust low surfaces

Preschoolers (3-5 years):
- Put away dishes
- Sweep floors
- Help with laundry (sorting, folding)
- Water plants
- Feed pets (with supervision)

Elementary School (6-9 years):
- Make their bed
- Set the table
- Help with meal preparation
- Take out the trash
- Vacuum
- Sweep
- Weed the garden

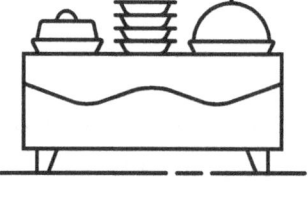

Older Children (10-12 years):
- Do laundry
- Load and unload the dishwasher
- Clean the bathroom
- Help with grocery shopping
- Mow the lawn
- Babysit younger siblings (with adult supervision)

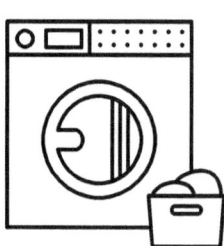

Remember to:

Start small: Begin with simple tasks and gradually increase responsibilities.
Be positive: Offer praise and encouragement.
Make it fun: Turn chores into games or competitions.
Be flexible: Adjust chores based on individual abilities and interests.

By incorporating age-appropriate chores into your child's routine, you can help them develop valuable life skills and a sense of responsibility.

Sensory Bins

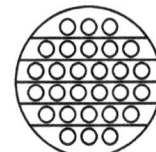

Sensory Bins: A Multi-Sensory Experience

Sensory bins offer a fun and engaging way for children to explore different textures and materials. Unlike traditional toys, sensory bins provide a variety of sensory experiences, stimulating both motor and sensory development.

Creating a Sensory Bin:

- **Safety first:** Avoid small objects for young children or those who put items in their mouths.
- **Consider allergies:** Be mindful of common allergens like red dyes, gluten, and latex.
- **Prevent overstimulation:** For children seeking tactile input or with visual seeking behavior, start with a limited number of items and gradually add more as tolerated.

Sensory bin materials can be purchased or homemade. Experiment with different materials to find what works best for your child. Remember to prioritize safety and consider individual needs when creating your sensory bin.

Here are some ideas to get you started:

1. **Dry Rice or Pasta:** These are great base materials. You can dye them with food coloring to make them more visually appealing.
2. **Water Beads:** These tiny beads expand in water and offer a unique texture experience. Ensure they are kept away from young children who might swallow them.
3. **Sand:** Kinetic sand is particularly popular because it sticks to itself and is less messy than traditional sand.
4. **Beans or Lentils:** These provide a satisfying crunch and can be used for scooping and pouring activities.
5. **Nature Items:** Incorporate pinecones, leaves, shells, and stones to bring an element of the outdoors inside.
6. **Slime or Oobleck:** These materials are great for kids who love messy play. They can be made at home with common household ingredients.

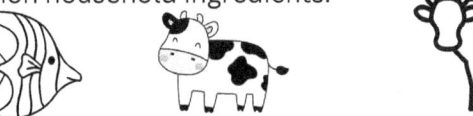

Themed Sensory Bins:

1. **Under the Sea:** Use blue-dyed rice or water beads, plastic sea creatures, and shells.
2. **Construction Site:** Fill with kinetic sand, toy trucks, and small rocks.
3. **Farmyard Fun:** Include dried corn kernels, plastic farm animals, and mini tractors.
4. **Arctic Adventure:** White rice or cotton balls can mimic snow, and add plastic polar animals and ice cubes for a chilly touch.

  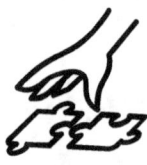

Engagement Tips:

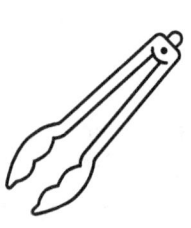

- **Storytelling:** Pair the sensory bin with a story or themed books to enhance the imaginative experience.
- **Tools:** Provide scoops, tongs, and containers to encourage fine motor skills development.
- **Observation:** Watch how your child interacts with different materials to gauge their preferences and comfort levels.

Maintaining Sensory Bins:

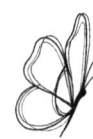

- **Cleanliness:** Clean and sanitize the materials periodically to ensure they remain safe for play.
- **Rotation:** Rotate toys and materials to keep the sensory bin fresh and exciting.
- **Storage:** Store items in clear containers to make setup and cleanup easy.

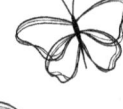
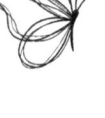

Sensory bins not only provide hours of entertainment but also support a child's development in numerous ways. They encourage exploration, creativity, and learning through play, making them a valuable addition to any playtime routine.

When working with very young children or those who tend to put objects in their mouths, opt for food items to avoid any allergy concerns. Some engaging options are cool whip, cooked noodles, jellies and jams, flour, and cornmeal.

Environmental Modifications: Creating a Sensory-Friendly Space

The environment plays a significant role in children's development and behavior, especially for those with sensory processing concerns, anxiety, ADHD, or trauma.

Furniture Safety and Organization:

- **Stability:** Ensure furniture is sturdy to prevent tip-overs.
- **Space:** Avoid overcrowding to provide ample room for movement.
- **Organization:** Declutter and use labels to designate specific areas for items.

Sensory Considerations:

- **Visual distractions:** Minimize wall, floor, and ceiling decorations to reduce visual overload.
- **Auditory stimulation:** Consider noise-reducing materials and limit background noise.
- **Olfactory sensitivity:** Choose non-toxic materials and avoid strong odors.
- **Tactile experiences:** Provide opportunities for sensory exploration through textures and materials.

Environmental Modifications:
- The environment significantly impacts children with sensory processing issues, anxiety, ADHD, and trauma.
- Besides visual aspects, consider auditory and olfactory stimuli when assessing the environment.

Decorations:
- **Limit** wall, floor, and ceiling decorations to avoid visual distractions and overwhelm.
- **Prioritize** safety considerations, like preventing climbing on furniture or accessing items that can be pulled off the walls.

Organization:
- **Clutter** can lead to chaos and confusion, so establish designated spaces for items to maintain order.
- Use **visual labels** to indicate where items belong, and consider organizing toys and games in cubbies and small containers for easy access and tidiness.

Create a Calming Atmosphere

- **Soft lighting:** Use warm-toned lighting to create a soothing ambiance.
- **Natural elements:** Incorporate plants or natural materials for a calming effect.
- **Quiet zones:** Designate specific areas for relaxation and sensory breaks.

By addressing these environmental factors, you can create a more supportive and inclusive space for children with sensory processing needs.

Furniture Safety and Organization:

- **Sturdy furniture:** Ensure furniture is secure and stable to prevent tip-overs.
- **Avoid overcrowding:** Provide ample floor space for play.
- **Consider sensory sensitivities:** Minimize visual, auditory, and olfactory distractions.
- **Safety first:** Assess potential hazards like climbing on shelves or reaching items on walls.
- **Organization:** Declutter the space and use labels to designate specific areas for items.

A well-organized and minimally cluttered environment can significantly impact children with sensory processing concerns, anxiety, ADHD, and trauma. By creating a calm and predictable space, you can help reduce stress and promote positive behavior.

Involving Children in Organization:
- **Empowerment:** Allow children to participate in organizing their space.
- **Ownership:** Foster a sense of responsibility for their belongings.
- **Educational opportunities:** Turn organization into a learning experience.

Creating a Calming Environment:

- **Soft lighting:** Use gentle lighting to create a soothing atmosphere.
- **Natural elements:** Incorporate plants to bring nature indoors.
- **Sensory stimulation:** Regularly rotate toys and activities to maintain interest and avoid overstimulation.
- **Quiet zones:** Designate specific areas for children to retreat when they need a break.

For children with anxiety or trauma:

- **Calming colors:** Use colors that promote relaxation.
- **Consistent routines:** Establish predictable schedules and rules.

By thoughtfully designing the environment, you can create a safe, focused, and supportive space that fosters children's growth and well-being.

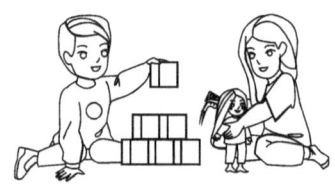

Variety of Lighting Options:

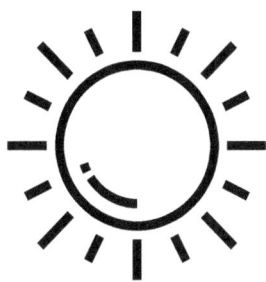

Types of Lightning

- **Adjustable lighting:** Dimmers, adjustable lamps, and overhead lighting with multiple settings provide flexibility and control.
- **Natural light:** Incorporate windows and skylights to maximize exposure to natural light.
- **Color-changing LED lights:** Add vibrancy and variety to the space.
- **Reminder:** Be cautious with lamps to prevent them from being easily knocked over, especially if they are within a child's reach.

Benefits of Natural and Artificial Lighting:

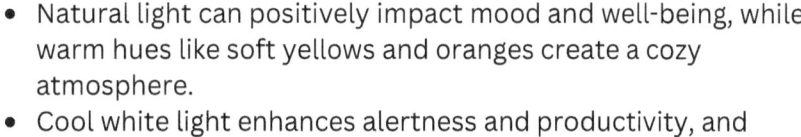

- Natural light can positively impact mood and well-being, while warm hues like soft yellows and oranges create a cozy atmosphere.
- Cool white light enhances alertness and productivity, and exposure to natural light helps regulate children's circadian rhythm for a healthy sleep cycle.
- Bright, evenly distributed light reduces eye strain and fatigue, aiding children in focusing on tasks and absorbing information effectively.
- Natural light positively affects mood, enhancing happiness and overall well-being.
- Warm lighting tones like soft yellows and oranges create a cozy ambiance.
- Artificial lighting is crucial but should not replace natural light.
- Including windows and skylights in educational spaces offers health benefits like improved mood, vitamin D synthesis, and enhanced well-being.

Effects of Different Lighting Types:

- **Blue-enriched light** boosts alertness and attention, ideal for tasks requiring focus, whereas warmer tones promote relaxation, beneficial for creative thinking.
- **Properly positioned** light sources in **educational settings** reduce glare and shadows, improving visual perception and learning experience.
- **Warmer tones** encourage relaxation, aiding creative thinking and problem-solving.

Incorporating Natural Light and Colorful Lighting:

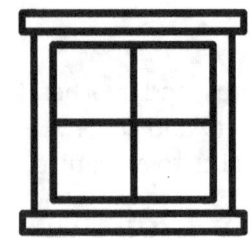

- Incorporate **windows and skylights** for natural light benefits, including improved mood and overall well-being.
- Color-changing LED lights and colorful fixtures can enhance the environment, **offering flexibility** for various activities and moods.
- Exposure to natural light **helps regulate** children's circadian rhythm, crucial for a healthy sleep-wake cycle, impacting mood, behavior, and cognitive development.

Importance of Adjustable Lighting:

- Provide lighting options that can be **easily adjusted** to accommodate different tasks and preferences.
- Adjustable lighting **supports children's activities** throughout the day, promoting comfort and control in their spaces.
- It caters to **sensory sensitivities** and **visual impairments**, ensuring inclusivity and accessibility for all children.

The Psychology of Color in Child Development

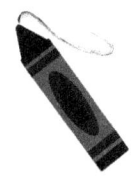

Red:

- Encourages energy and excitement in children.
- Might prompt kids to stay active.
- Excessive red can be overwhelming or distracting.
- Not ideal for spaces where focus or relaxation is needed, like bedrooms or classrooms.

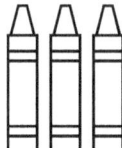

Orange:

- Encourages social interaction.
- Evokes feelings of happiness and enthusiasm.
- Seeing orange in the morning can boost kids' alertness.
- Great for rooms that foster creativity and friendship.

Yellow:

- Instills joy, laughter, kindness, and wisdom.
- May enhance concentration and memory.
- Too much yellow or intense shades can lead to anger and frustration.

Green:

- Improves children's concentration and reading comprehension.
- Associated with safety and positivity.
- Ideal for bedroom decor to aid faster sleep

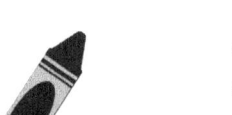

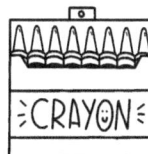

Blue:

- Known for its calming effects.
- Helps children relax and unwind.
- A blue environment can lower heart rate and blood pressure.
- Excessive dark blue may heighten anxiety and depression.

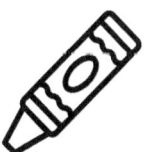

Purple:

- Boosts creativity and overall well-being.
- Has a calming influence, aiding emotional development and imagination.

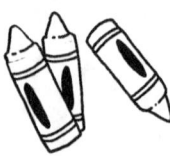

Pink:

- Similar to blue, pink lowers heart rate.
- Considered soothing and comfortable.
- Overuse may overwhelm shy or introverted children.

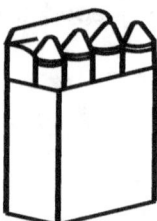

Brown:

- Represents stability and reliability, grounding children.

Black:

- Offers some children a sense of equilibrium.
- Too much black can be overwhelming or frightening.

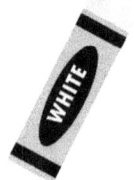

White:

- Acts as a neutral color, balancing darker tones.
- Excessive white can stifle creativity and learning.

When designing children's spaces, consider the following:

Balance: Combine neutral colors with subtle pops of brighter hues.
Individual preferences: Observe how your child responds to different colors.
Purpose of the space: Choose colors that align with the room's function (e.g., calming colors for bedrooms, stimulating colors for play areas)

Remember, while colors can influence behavior, individual preferences and sensitivities vary. It's essential to create a space that is comfortable and supportive for your child.

Safety

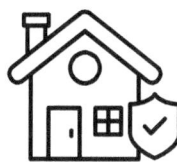

Safety Measures for Children
Some children have a tendency to run away or hide, which can be risky and frightening. It is crucial to plan and be prepared.

At Home:

- **Doors and window alarms** can be found at most major department stores and are simple to set up. Using a wooden dowel to secure sliding doors and windows is a cost-effective option.
- **Refrigerator alarms and locks** are also easily accessible. If your child tends to hide, ensure that the washer and dryer are not easily reachable. Large coolers and suitcases are potential hiding spots where a child might get stuck. If your child enjoys climbing, be cautious of climbing on the stove. Stove knobs can be removed or covered to prevent accidental climbing and burns.
- **Plug covers and light switch covers** can prevent children from touching electrical outlets or constantly switching lights on and off.

Car Seats:

- Many children can **unbuckle** their car seat. Car seat buckle covers are available to enhance car seat safety.
- **Ensure** the car seat is properly installed and that the harness is snug but comfortable. Regularly check the car seat for wear and tear, and replace it as needed.

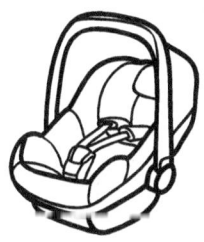

In Public:

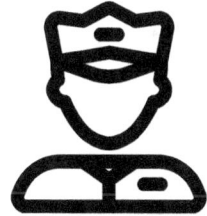

- **Establish a safety plan** with your child, such as knowing their full name, your phone number, and what to do if they get separated from you. Utilize identification bracelets or tags with your contact information.
- **Teach your child** about the importance of staying close to you and holding hands in crowded places. Point out safe adults, like police officers or store employees, whom they can approach if they need help.
- **Use safety harnesses or wristbands** if your child is prone to wandering. These can provide an extra layer of security while allowing your child some freedom to explore.

Online Safety:

- Monitor your child's online activity and use parental controls to restrict access to inappropriate content. Educate them about the dangers of sharing personal information online.
- Set clear rules about screen time and ensure that your child understands the importance of privacy and the potential risks of interacting with strangers on the internet.

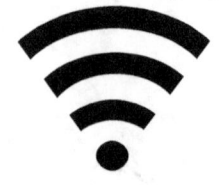

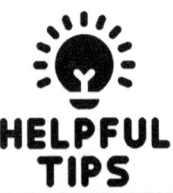

General Tips:

- Keep a recent photo of your child and their medical information handy, in case of an emergency.
- Teach your child about basic safety rules, such as not talking to strangers, looking both ways before crossing the street, and understanding what to do in case of a fire or other emergencies.

By implementing these safety measures, you can create a more secure environment for your child, minimizing risks and providing peace of mind for the entire family.

Nurturing Your Babies Brain Development and Fostering Co-Regulation Strategies

Nurturing Your Baby's Brain Development

To foster your baby's brain development, prioritize the following:

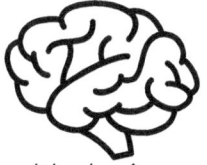

- **Love and attention:** Responsive care builds trust and security, promoting healthy brain connections.
- **Positive experiences:** Engage your baby through interactions, smiles, songs, and cuddles.
- **Stimulating activities:** Play, talk, read, and sing to provide enriching experiences.
- **Calm and loving environment:** A peaceful home promotes your baby's emotional well-being.
- **Consistent routines:** Predictable schedules create a sense of security.
- **Healthy nutrition:** Breast milk or formula provides essential nutrients for brain development.
- **Regular check-ups:** Ensure that your baby attends all recommended pediatric visits to monitor growth and development milestones.
  - Early detection of any potential issues can lead to timely interventions.
- **Safe sleep practices:** Always place your baby on their back to sleep, in a crib free from soft bedding and toys, to reduce the risk of Sudden Infant Death Syndrome (SIDS).
- **Social interaction:** Encourage playdates and interactions with other children to help develop social skills.
  - Even simple activities like face-to-face play and mirroring expressions can be beneficial.
- **Physical activity:** Allow your baby to have plenty of tummy time and opportunities to explore their environment.
  - This supports motor skills development and spatial awareness.
- **Limit screen time:** Avoid exposing your baby to screens such as televisions, tablets, or smartphones.
  - Instead, focus on direct human interaction, which is far more beneficial at this stage.
- **Parental well-being:** Take care of yourself, too. Your mental and physical health directly impacts your ability to provide the best care for your baby. Seek support when needed, and make time for self-care

By integrating these practices into your daily routine, you are creating a nurturing and stimulating environment that supports your baby's holistic development, laying a strong foundation for their future learning and growth.

Remember, these simple steps can significantly impact your baby's cognitive growth and future development.

Self Regulation and Co-Regulation Strategies

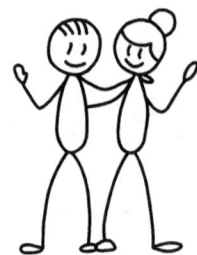

Strategies for Adults :

- **Keep Calm:** Children mirror the emotional state of adults. Staying composed can help the child manage their own emotions. Take deep breaths, speak soothingly, and maintain a gentle expression.

- **Acknowledge Their Feelings:** Validate the child's emotions, even if you don't approve of their actions. Phrases like "I understand you're frustrated" or "It's okay to feel angry" can make them feel heard.

- **Provide Physical Comfort:** Sometimes, a hug, holding their hand, or staying close can make a child feel safe. Respect their comfort level with physical touch.

- **Demonstrate Calming Techniques:** Practice deep breathing, counting, or gentle stretches together. Showing how you calm down can teach the child to do the same.

- **Reduce Distractions:** Excessive stimuli can overwhelm during emotional moments. If possible, move the child away from the trigger and find a quiet space.

- **Use Simple Language:** Speak clearly and calmly, avoiding complex explanations. Focus on the present moment to help the child understand.

Establish Clear Boundaries: While validating emotions, set firm but respectful boundaries for behavior. Communicate what is acceptable in a way that suits the child's age.

Seek Professional Help if Needed: If an adult or child consistently struggles with intense emotions or behavior, it might be beneficial to seek help from a psychologist or counselor. Professional support can provide additional strategies and insights to help both the child and the adult.

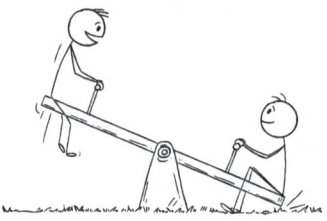

Strategies for the Child:

- **Sensory Activities:** Provide calming sensory activities such as fidget toys, play dough, squeezing a stress ball, or deep pressure massages. These can offer a sense of relief and help the child focus their energy.

- **Movement:** Movement can be a great way for children to release pent-up emotions. Activities like jumping, dancing, or going for a walk can be helpful.

- **Breathing Exercises:** Teach the child simple breathing exercises like slow, deep belly breaths. This can help slow their heart rate and calm their nervous system.

- **Mindfulness Techniques:** If the child is old enough, introduce simple mindfulness techniques like focusing on their breath or counting their calming thoughts.

- **Positive Reinforcement:** When the child is able to self-regulate, acknowledge their progress and offer praise. This will encourage them to continue using these strategies in the future.

Additional Tips:

- **Be Patient:** Co-regulation takes time and practice. Be patient with yourself and the child, and celebrate even small successes.

- **Consistency is Key:** Consistency in your approach will help the child learn what to expect and feel more secure.

- **Age-Appropriate Strategies:** The specific strategies you use will vary depending on the child's age and developmental stage.

- **Seek Professional Help:** If you're struggling to co-regulate with your child, consider seeking professional help from a therapist or counselor who specializes in child development.

Behavior Tracker

Complete the tracker for at least 3 days. The longer you track and gather information, the more insightful your data will become.

- **Time:** What time of day did the behavior occur?

- **Behavior:**
    - What did the child do?
    - Did the child scream, kick, run, hit or throw?

- **Length of time:**
    - How long did the behavior last?

- **What happened before and who was present.** Think about the sensory environment.
    - Was it hot? Did it smell different?
    - Was there a loud noise?
    - Were the lights dim or bright?
    - Were there people around that the child was not familiar with?

- **What stopped the behavior:**
    - Were you able to redirect?
    - Did a hug stop the behavior?

Behavior Tracker

Complete the tracker for at least 3 days. The longer you track and gather information, the more insightful your data will become.

Time of day	Behavior	Length of time	What happened before the incident and who was present	What stopped the behavior

Strategies and Diagnosis

Outlined below are the diagnoses and concerns, along with strategies that may be helpful. **Remember these are mere suggestions and should not replace advice given by your child's medical professional.**

Strategies	Anxiety	Depression	ADHD	Sleep	Autism
Schedules	X		X	X	X
Video Modeling			X		X
Personal Stories	X	X	X	X	X
Daily Report Card			X		X
Weighted Vest					X
Weighted Blanket	X			X	X
Lycra Sheets	X			X	X
Music	X	X	X	X	X
Noise Cancelling Headphones					X

Always consult with a healthcare provider to ensure that your child receives the appropriate care tailored to their unique needs.

Consider keeping a journal to track any changes or concerns, and don't hesitate to ask questions during medical appointments.

Strategies	Sensory Motor	Sensory Modulation Tactile	Sensory Modulation Auditory	Sensory Modulation Proprioception	Sensory Modulation Vestibular
Schedules	X				
Video Modeling	X				
Personal Stories	X	X	X	X	X
Daily Report Card					
Weighted Vest				X	
Weighted Blanket				X	
Lycra Sheets				X	
Music	X		X		
Noise Cancelling Headphones			X		

RESOURCES

Disclaimer: This list of resources is not exhaustive and is intended for informational purposes only. For a comprehensive list of resources and personalized guidance, please consult with a healthcare professional or specialist in the field of Autism, ADHD, Trauma or Sensory Processing disorders.

GENERAL RESOURCES

Brewer Educational Resources
https://brewerlearningcatalog.com/
Brewer Educational Resources is dedicated to educational resources and professional development for educators.

Celebrate Successful Early Learning
https://celebratesel.com/
This is a website that sells products designed to teach young children early literacy skills, such as reading, writing, and math. The products use fun and engaging techniques, like songs, rhymes, and repetition, to keep children interested. They are also available in both English and Spanish.

Child Therapy Toys
https://www.childtherapytoys.com/
Child therapy toys are specially designed tools that can be used by therapists to help children express their emotions, process traumatic experiences, and develop coping skills.

Child's Play
https://childsplaybooks.myshopify.com/
Child's Play is a popular children's book popular book publisher known for its engaging stories, colorful illustrations, and educational value. Books available in Spanish/English Bilingual.

Fun and Function
http://funandfunction.com/
Designs special needs toys, autism toys, and therapy products ideal for occupational therapy activities for children

GENERAL RESOURCES

Kaplan Learning Co.
https://www.kaplanco.com/
Kaplan Early Learning Company is a website that sells educational products and services for early childhood classrooms. They offer a variety of furniture, playground equipment, art supplies, and other classroom essentials. Additionally, they provide curriculum and professional development resources.

Learning Resources
https://www.learningresources.com/
Learning Resources.com is a website and company that provides educational toys, games, and classroom materials for children of all ages, with a focus on early childhood education.

Pocket full of Therapy
http://www.pfot.com/
Sells weighted blankets, desk buddy, organizational pouches for school chairs, and so on

Therapy Shoppe
http://www.therapyshoppe.com/
Sells large variety of products including slant boards, therapy balls, and weighted vests.

ADHD- Attention Deficit Disorder Resources

Children and Adults with Attention-Deficit/Hyperactivity Disorder (CHADD)
https://chadd.org/
CHADD is a nonprofit organization dedicated to improving the lives of individuals affected by ADHD. They provide education, advocacy, and support for people of all ages with ADHD and their families.

The ADDitude Magazine
https://www.additudemag.com/
ADDitude Magazine is a leading resource for individuals living with ADHD and their families. It provides comprehensive information, advice, and support on various aspects of ADHD.

ADHD- Attention Deficit Disorder Resources

Children and Adults with Attention-Deficit/Hyperactivity Disorder (CHADD)
https://chadd.org/
CHADD is a nonprofit organization dedicated to improving the lives of individuals affected by ADHD. They provide education, advocacy, and support for people of all ages with ADHD and their families.

ADHD- Attention Deficit Disorder Resources

Children and Adults with Attention-Deficit/Hyperactivity Disorder (CHADD)
https://chadd.org/
CHADD is a nonprofit organization dedicated to improving the lives of individuals affected by ADHD. They provide education, advocacy, and support for people of all ages with ADHD and their families.

The ADDitude Magazine
https://www.additudemag.com/
ADDitude Magazine is a leading resource for individuals living with ADHD and their families. It provides comprehensive information, advice, and support on various aspects of ADHD.

Autism

Autism Research Institute
www.autism.com
Dedicated to the research and education on the causes of autism and on methods of preventing, diagnosing, and treating autism.

Autism Society of America
301-657-0881
www.autism-society.org
Leading source of information on autism

Autism Speaks
888-AUTISM2
www.autismspeaks.org
One of the largest foundations in the world solely dedicated to autism.

Developmental Delay Resources
www.devdelay.org
DDR is dedicated to meeting the needs of children with developmental delays in sensory, motor, language, social, and emotional areas.

The National Autism Association
877.622.2884
https://nationalautismassociation.org/
The National Autism Association's Big Red Safety Box® is a free-of-charge safety toolkit for autism families in need of wandering-prevention tools.

DIAGNOSIS-SPECIFIC INFORMATION

CDC-The Centers for Disease Control and Prevention
800-CDC-INFO (800-232-4636)
http://www.cdc.gov/Features/adhdresources/

National Organization for Rare Disorders (NORD)
https://rarediseases.org/
The National Organization for Rare Disorders (NORD) is a leading non-profit organization dedicated to supporting individuals and families affected by rare diseases. A rare disease is typically defined as a condition that affects a small number of people in a population.

Nutrition

Academy of Nutrition and Dietetics
https://www.eatright.org/
The Academy of Nutrition and Dietetics offers information on nutrition and health, from meal planning and prep to choices that can help prevent or manage health conditions and more.

Professional Development and Training

The National Association for the Education of Young Children (NAEYC)
https://www.naeyc.org/
The National Association for the Education of Young Children (NAEYC) is a leading organization in the United States dedicated to improving the well-being and education of young children, from birth to age 8.

Professional Development and Training

Division for Early Childhood
https://www.dec-sped.org/
The Division for Early Childhood (DEC) is a division of the Council for Exceptional Children (CEC), a global professional organization dedicated to improving educational outcomes for individuals with disabilities. DEC specifically focuses on children birth through age eight and their families.

Sensory Processing Disorder (SPD)

Sensory Processing Disorder Foundation
303-221-STAR (7827)
https://sensoryhealth.org/

Sensory Processing Disorder (SPD)

The Sensory Processing Disorder Resource Center
https://www.sensory-processing-disorder.com/

Sensory Processing Disorder Support Group
https://www.facebook.com/groups/sensoryplanet/
This group is comprised primarily of parents who are raising children with SPD.

Trauma

ATTACh
https://attach.org/
ATTACh is an international coalition dedicated to promoting awareness of trauma and attachment disorders in children and teens, and empowering caregivers and professionals to help them heal.

Child Therapy Toys
https://www.childtherapytoys.com/
Child therapy toys are specially designed tools that can be used by therapists to help children express their emotions, process traumatic experiences, and develop coping skills.

VIDEO MODELING/SOCIAL SKILLS VIDEOS

Model Me Kids
www.modelmekids.com/
Demonstrate social skills by modeling peer behavior at school, on a playdate, at a birthday party, on the playground, at a library, at the dentist, at a restaurant, and more. Designed as a teaching tool for children, adolescents, and teenagers with autism, Asperger syndrome, and developmental delays, the videos are used by teachers, parents, and therapists. Real children model each skill.

Social Skill Builders
www.socialskillbuilder.com/
Social Skill Builder's curriculum of researched-based, evidence-driven software programs use systematic and explicit instruction through interactive videos to teach key social thinking, language, and behavior that are critical to everyday living.

TV Teacher
www.tvteachervideos.com/contact
Developed by an occupational therapist who performs video-modeling programs to special-needs classes for handwriting and fine motor skills. All students can use this program for assistance with handwriting.

References

(2009, December 31). Occupational Therapy in School Settings. Www.aota.org.

American Physical Therapy Association (APTA). Physical Therapy in School Settings. Accessed at www.apta.org/uploadedFiles/APTAorg/Advocacy/Federal/Legislative_Issues/IDEA_ESEA/Physical TherapyintheSchoolSystem.pdf.

American Psychiatric Association. Diagnostic and Statistical Manual of Mental Disorders. 5th edition. Arlington, VA: American Psychiatric Association, 2013. Print.

Ayres, Jean. Sensory Integration and the Child: 25th Anniversary Edition. Torrance, CA: Western Psychological Services, April 1, 2005. Print.

Barkley, R. A. Fact Sheet: Attention Deficit Hyperactivity Disorder (ADHD) Topics. https://www.russellbarkley.org/factsheets/adhd-facts.pdf

Benson, Mary T. Parent Fact Sheet: Signs and Symptoms of Sensory Processing Disorder. Newton: The Spiral Foundation, 2006. Print.

Hyche, K., OTD, & Maertz, V., OTD (2014). Classroom Strategies For Children with ADHD, Autism & Sensory Processing Disorders: Solutions for Behavior, Attention and Emotional Regulation. Pesi.

Krouse, L. (2023, October 21). ADHD Criteria for Diagnosis Attention Deficit Hyperactivity Disorder in Adults and Children. Verywellhealth. https://www.verywellhealth.com/adhd-diagnosis

Yang FN, Xie W, Wang Z. Effects of sleep duration on neurocognitive development in early adolescents in the USA: a propensity score matched, longitudinal, observational study. Lancet Child Adolesc Health. 2022 Oct;6(10):705-712. doi: 10.1016/S2352-4642(22)00188-2. Epub 2022 Jul 30. PMID: 35914537; PMCID: PMC9482948.

Visit us @

for more information on each chapter

www.ingramcontent.com/pod-product-compliance
Lightning Source LLC
Chambersburg PA
CBHW062217220526
45471CB00009B/3237